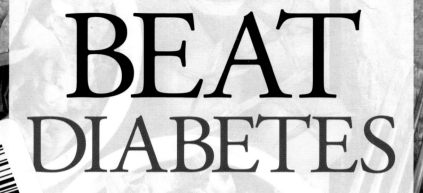

BEAT
DIABETES

5 Hints, Tips & Recipes

pil

Publications International, Ltd.

Goals for the year:

_____

_____

_____

_____

January 1

Take some time to reflect during the early days of the year—what are your goals this year for managing your diabetes? Are there any changes you want to make that will help you control your blood sugar, manage your diet, or add more movement to your life?

Many times, resolutions we make for ourselves in January are forgotten by February. So set yourself up for success! Keep your goals concrete, make sure they're sustainable, and start with small, achievable steps.

Metric Conversion Chart

BAKING PAN SIZES

UTENSIL	SIZE IN INCHES/QUARTS	METRIC VOLUME	SIZE IN CENTIMETERS
Baking or Cake Pan (square or rectangular)	8 × 8 × 2	2 L	20 × 20 × 5
	9 × 9 × 2	2.5 L	23 × 23 × 5
	12 × 8 × 2	3 L	30 × 20 × 5
	13 × 9 × 2	3.5 L	33 × 23 × 5
Loaf Pan	8 × 4 × 3	1.5 L	20 × 10 × 7
	9 × 5 × 3	2 L	23 × 13 × 7
Round Layer Cake Pan	8 × 1½	1.2 L	20 × 4
	9 × 1½	1.5 L	23 × 4
Pie Plate	8 × 1¼	750 mL	20 × 3
	9 × 1¼	1 L	23 × 3
Baking Dish or Casserole	1 quart	1 L	––
	1½ quart	1.5 L	––
	2 quart	2 L	––

OVEN TEMPERATURES

250°F = 120°C
275°F = 140°C
300°F = 150°C
325°F = 160°C
350°F = 180°C
375°F = 190°C
400°F = 200°C
425°F = 220°C
450°F = 230°C

DIMENSIONS

1/16 inch = 2 mm
1/8 inch = 3 mm
1/4 inch = 6 mm
1/2 inch = 1.5 cm
3/4 inch = 2 cm
1 inch = 2.5 cm

January 2

In our busy lives, it's easy to let things slip through the cracks...like routine checkups with the eye doctor. People with diabetes are at risk for diabetic retinopathy and other eye problems, but early diagnosis and intervention can help. Make a note on your calendar to schedule an annual appointment with your eye doctor.

Metric Conversion Chart

VOLUME MEASUREMENTS (dry)

⅛ teaspoon = 0.5 mL

¼ teaspoon = 1 mL

½ teaspoon = 2 mL

¾ teaspoon = 4 mL

1 teaspoon = 5 mL

1 tablespoon = 15 mL

2 tablespoons = 30 mL

¼ cup = 60 mL

⅓ cup = 75 mL

½ cup = 125 mL

⅔ cup = 150 mL

¾ cup = 175 mL

1 cup = 250 mL

2 cups = 1 pint = 500 mL

3 cups = 750 mL

4 cups = 1 quart = 1 L

VOLUME MEASUREMENTS (fluid)

1 fluid ounce (2 tablespoons) = 30 mL

4 fluid ounces (½ cup) = 125 mL

8 fluid ounces (1 cup) = 250 mL

12 fluid ounces (1½ cups) = 375 mL

16 fluid ounces (2 cups) = 500 mL

WEIGHTS (MASS)

½ ounce = 15 g

1 ounce = 30 g

3 ounces = 90 g

4 ounces = 120 g

8 ounces = 225 g

10 ounces = 285 g

12 ounces = 360 g

16 ounces = 1 pound = 450 g

4 teaspoons vegetable oil-and-yogurt spread
8 slices whole grain cinnamon raisin bread
¼ cup reduced-fat cream cheese
¼ cup low-sugar red raspberry preserves

1 medium Granny Smith apple
  (about 5 ounces), thinly sliced
⅛ teaspoon ground cinnamon

1. Spread ½ teaspoon spread onto one side of bread slices. Spread 1 tablespoon cream cheese on opposite side of four bread slices. Arrange apple slices over cream cheese. Spread 1 tablespoon preserves on opposite side of remaining four bread slices; sprinkle with cinnamon. Place on top of apples to create sandwich.

2. Coat large nonstick skillet with nonstick cooking spray; heat over medium heat. Grill sandwiches 2 to 3 minutes on each side or until golden brown.

Makes 4 servings

Dietary Exchanges: 2½ Starch, 1 Fat

Calories 265, **Total Fat** 8g, **Saturated Fat** 3g, **Protein** 8g, **Carbohydrate** 36g, **Cholesterol** 10mg, **Dietary Fiber** 3g, **Sodium** 300mg

Places to Go

American Diabetes Association:
www.diabetes.org

American Heart Association:
www.heart.org

Centers for Disease Control and Prevention,
Diabetes Public Health Resource:
www.cdc.gov/diabetes

Joslin Diabetes Center:
www.joslin.org

National Diabetes Information Clearinghouse
diabetes.niddk.nih.gov

January 4

Diabetes has been around for a long time. Papyrus documents from ancient Egypt, were written about 3,500 years ago, appear to be medical records that describe patients with the symptoms of diabetes.

Notes

January 5

Stressed out? When your stress levels increase, so do your blood pressure, heart rate, and blood sugar level.

It can help just to identify the causes of stress in your life. Think through strategies for dealing with frequent stressors ahead of time, when you're calm.

Name of Optometrist/ Ophthalmologist	Date	Purpose of Visit
_____	_____	_____
_____	_____	_____
_____	_____	_____
_____	_____	_____
_____	_____	_____
_____	_____	_____
_____	_____	_____
_____	_____	_____

January 6

Although kale can be found year around, it is at its best when the weather is cooler. This nutritional powerhouse is packed with vitamins A, C, K, and B6. Steamed kale in particular provides a lot of health benefits, such as increased protection against cancer.

Dentist's Name	Date	Purpose of Visit

1 small onion, chopped
3 slices turkey bacon, chopped
4 cups coarsely chopped kale leaves
2 cloves garlic, minced
2 cups cholesterol-free egg substitute

¼ teaspoon ground black pepper
¼ teaspoon salt (optional)
1 container (4 ounces) crumbled
   goat cheese

1. Spray large ovenproof skillet with cooking spray; heat over medium heat. Add onion and bacon; cook and stir 6 to 8 minutes or until onion is light golden.

2. Add kale and garlic; cook 3 to 5 minutes or until kale is wilted. Evenly spread mixture to cover bottom of skillet.

3. Whisk egg substitute, pepper and salt, if desired in small bowl until well blended. Pour evenly over kale mixture; sprinkle evenly with cheese. Cover and cook 6 to 7 minutes or until almost set.

4. Preheat broiler. Uncover skillet; broil 2 to 3 minutes or until golden brown and set. Let stand 5 minutes before cutting into 6 wedges.

Makes 6 servings

Dietary Exchanges: ½ Fat, 1 Vegetable, 1½ Meat

Calories 120, **Total Fat** 6g, **Saturated Fat** 3g, **Protein** 13g, **Carbohydrates** 5g, **Cholesterol** 25mg, **Dietary Fiber** 1g, **Sodium** 320mg

Doctor's Name	Date	Purpose of Visit

January 8

Quick Quiz

How many people have diabetes worldwide?

    A. About 20 to 30 million
    B. About 100 to 120 million
    C. About 340 to 350 million
    D. 1 billion

Answer: C. In the United States alone, there are about 29 million people with diabetes.

Doctor's Name	Date	Purpose of Visit
_____	_____	_____
_____	_____	_____
_____	_____	_____
_____	_____	_____
_____	_____	_____
_____	_____	_____
_____	_____	_____
_____	_____	_____

January 9

Staying active in winter can be difficult. Here are just a few ways you can keep moving, whatever the weather:

- Get a membership to a museum where you can walk while looking at exhibits.

- Check whether any local facilities have heated indoor swimming pools.

- Join a social dancing class through your local park district or community center. Or just clear some floor space at home and turn up the music!

Doctor's Name	Date	Purpose of Visit
_____	_____	_____
_____	_____	_____
_____	_____	_____
_____	_____	_____
_____	_____	_____
_____	_____	_____
_____	_____	_____
_____	_____	_____

1 pound boneless skinless chicken breasts, cooked

1 cup chopped broccoli

1 cup diced carrots

1 can (10¾ ounces) 98% fat-free condensed
cream of celery soup, undiluted

¼ cup reduced-fat (2%) milk

1 tablespoon dry sherry

½ cup grated Parmesan cheese

6 (10-inch) fat-free flour tortilla

1. Preheat oven to 350°F. Spray 13×9-inch baking dish with nonstick cooking spray; set aside. Cut chicken into 1-inch pieces; set aside.

2. Combine broccoli and carrots in 1-quart microwavable dish. Cover and microwave on HIGH 2 to 3 minutes or until vegetables are crisp-tender; set aside.

3. Combine soup, milk and sherry in small saucepan over medium heat; cook and stir 5 minutes. Stir in Parmesan cheese, chicken, broccoli and carrots. Cook 2 minutes or until cheese is melted. Remove from heat.

4. Spoon ¼ cup chicken mixture onto each tortilla. Roll up and place, seam side down, in prepared baking dish. Bake, covered, 20 minutes or until heated through.

Makes 6 servings

Dietary Exchanges: 2 Bread/Starch, 1 Vegetable, 2 Meat

Calories 284, **Total Fat** 5g, **Saturated Fat** 2g, **Protein** 26g, **Carbohydrates** 33g, **Cholesterol** 52mg, **Dietary Fiber** 11g, **Sodium** 733mg

Glucagon Emergency Kit

If you take insulin or if you have hypoglycemia unawareness, keep a glucagon emergency kit on hand for severe hypoglycemic reactions. Make sure the people around you know where it is kept and are trained in its use.

The location of my glucagon emergency kit(s):

_____

_____

_____

_____

January 11

When your blood sugar is under control, it affects the whole of your body, including your gums. The lower your blood sugar level, the lower your risk of gum disease and tooth loss. Another step you can take to keep your teeth and gums healthy is to schedule regular cleanings and checkups with your dentist.

Fast-Acting Carbohydrates

15 grams of fast-acting carbohydrates can be found in the following foods.

3–4 glucose tabs
4 ounces of fruit juice
5 sugar cubes
1 small box of raisins
1 cup of skim milk
1 tablespoon of honey
6 hard candies

January 12

Did you know that Thomas Edison had diabetes? It didn't stop him from helping to shape the modern world—when he died in 1931 at the age of 84, the legendary inventor of the light bulb had over 1,000 patents to his name.

Addressing Hypoglycemia

If your blood glucose level drops beneath 70 mg/dl, or if you're experiencing symptoms of hypoglycemia, do the following:

1. Eat 15 grams of a fast-acting carbohydrate.
   (For examples, see the following page.)
2. Wait 15 minutes. Then, if you're able to check your blood glucose level, do so. If you don't have testing equipment available, are the symptoms still present?
3. If your blood glucose level is still low or you're still experiencing symptoms, eat another 15 grams of a fast-acting carbohydrate.
4. When the symptoms are gone, if it is more than one hour from a mealtime, eat a small snack that includes protein, fat, and carbohydrate.

January 13

Myth or Fact? If you have type 2 diabetes, your child has a greater chance of developing it.

Fact. Having a parent (or other close relative) with type 2 diabetes increases someone's risk of developing it themselves. If you have diabetes, encourage your children and other close family members to lead a healthy, active lifestyle that will help minimize their risk.

Later Symptoms of Hypoglycemia

Headache
Blurred vision
Slurred speech
Confusion
Euphoria
Hostility
Lack of coordination
Drowsiness
Convulsions
Loss of consciousness
For treatment, see the following page.

8 ounces uncooked whole wheat penne or rigatoni pasta

1½ cups frozen cut green beans

3 teaspoons olive oil, divided

3 green onions, sliced

1 clove garlic, minced

1 can (about 14 ounces) diced Italian-style tomatoes, drained

½ teaspoon salt

½ teaspoon Italian seasoning

¼ teaspoon black pepper

1 can (12 ounces) solid albacore tuna packed in water, drained and flaked

1. Cook pasta according to package directions, omitting salt and fat. Add green beans during last 7 minutes of cooking time (allow water to return to a boil before resuming timing). Drain and keep warm.

2. Meanwhile, heat 1 teaspoon oil in large skillet over medium heat. Cook and stir green onions and garlic 2 minutes. Add tomatoes, salt, Italian seasoning and pepper; cook and stir 4 to 5 minutes. Add pasta mixture, tuna and remaining 2 teaspoons oil; mix gently. Serve immediately.

Makes 6 Servings

Dietary Exchanges: 2 Bread/Starch, 1 Vegetable, 3 Meat

Calories 228, **Total Fat** 4g, **Saturated Fat** 1g, **Protein** 15g, **Carbohydrates** 34g, **Cholesterol** 14mg, **Dietary Fiber** 3g, **Sodium** 345mg

Early Symptoms of Hypoglycemia

Dizziness
Pale or flushed face
Irritability
Hunger
Sweating
Rapid heartbeat
Fatigue or weakness
Feelings of anxiety or nervousness
Shakiness
Queasiness
Headache

For later symptoms and treatment of hypoglycemia,
see the following pages.

January 15

There is no special "diabetic diet." While people with diabetes need to take special care in managing their blood sugar, they, their spouses or partners, and their families can all strive for a varied, heart-healthy diet that's full of tasty, colorful foods. To help your family members eat well, show them the easy-to-use plate method. At meals, about one-half of the plate should be full of non-starchy vegetables. Divide the other half of the plate equally between grains/starchy foods, protein, and fruit or dairy.

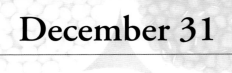

December 31

As the year closes, look back over your accomplishments. What steps have you taken this year that have helped you manage your diabetes or control your blood sugar? Celebrate the times you've made good choices, the habits from which you've benefited, and those people who have given you support along the way!

January 16

One way to teach your kids or grandkids how to incorporate good eating habits is to have them help you shop for and prepare meals. Encourage them to pick out a vegetable or fruit they've never tried before and introduce it to the family.

2 tablespoons whole wheat flour

2 tablespoons granulated sugar

1 tablespoon cocoa powder, plus additional for garnish

1½ to 2 teaspoons instant coffee granules

1 egg white

3 tablespoons fat-free (skim) milk

2 teaspoons mini semisweet chocolate chips

1 teaspoon vegetable oil

1 tablespoon thawed frozen fat-free whipped topping

1. Combine flour, sugar, 1 tablespoon cocoa powder and coffee granules in large ceramic* microwavable mug; mix well. Whisk egg white, milk and oil in small bowl until well blended. Stir into flour mixture until smooth. Fold in chocolate chips.

2. Microwave on HIGH 2 minutes. Let stand 1 to 2 minutes before serving. Top with whipped topping and additional cocoa, if desired.

A ceramic mug is necessary. The material allows for more even cooking than glass.

Makes 1 serving

Dietary Exchanges: 3 Bread/Starch, 1½ Fat

Calories 286, **Total Fat** 8g, **Saturated Fat** 2g, **Protein** 9g, **Carbohydrates** 50g, **Cholesterol** 1mg, **Dietary Fiber** 4g, **Sodium** 80mg

TOFU, VEGETABLE AND CURRY STIR-FRY

1 package (about 14 ounces) extra-firm reduced-fat tofu, cut into ¾-inch cubes

¾ cup reduced-fat coconut milk

2 tablespoons fresh lime juice

1 tablespoon curry powder

2 teaspoons dark sesame oil, divided

4 cups broccoli florets (1½ inch pieces)

2 medium red bell peppers, cut into short, thin strips

1 medium red onion, cut into thin wedges

¼ teaspoon salt

1. Press tofu cubes between layers of paper towels to remove excess moisture. Combine coconut milk, lime juice and curry powder in medium bowl.

2. Heat 1 teaspoon oil in large nonstick skillet over medium heat. Add tofu; cook 10 minutes or until lightly browned on all sides, turning cubes often. Remove to plate; set aside.

3. Add remaining 1 teaspoon oil to skillet; increase heat to high. Add broccoli, bell pepper and onion; stir-fry about 5 minutes or until vegetables are crisp-tender. Stir in tofu and coconut milk mixture; cook and stir until mixture comes to a boil. Stir in salt. Serve immediately.

Makes 4 servings

Dietary Exchanges: 1 Fat, 4 Vegetable, 1 Meat

Calories 167, **Total Fat** 8g, **Saturated Fat** 2g, **Protein** 12g, **Carbohydrates** 16g, **Cholesterol** 0mg, **Dietary Fiber** 5g, **Sodium** 159mg

December 29

Take some time to look back over any logbooks and food diaries you kept during the year. What patterns do you see? Can they help shape your goals for the coming year?

January 18

Staying active can become a family affair. If you're taking the dog out for a walk, invite along a family member. If your children are young, look into parent-child activity classes at your local park district or community center. Get a family membership to a local museum or botanic garden.

December 28

Because diabetes is a progressive disease, your diabetes program needs to be dynamic, changing with your individual needs—and with the progress that new technology, new research, and new treatments bring! Periodically examine the steps you're taking to manage your diabetes. Do those steps still give you optimal control? If not, it's time to make an appointment with your health care provider to try something new—an increased dose of insulin, or perhaps a different oral medication or a different dosage.

January 19

What Are Exchange Lists?

Exchange lists divide food into six categories: vegetables, milk, meat, fruit, starch, and fat. Foods in each group have similar amounts of carbohydrate, protein, and fat. If your meal plan calls for one starch exchange (15 grams carbohydrate) for breakfast, you can look at an exchange list to see that that's equivalent to ¾ cup cold cereal, half a frozen bagel, or 1 slice of whole-wheat bread.

1 package (about 18 ounces)
   yellow cake mix
¾ cup reduced-fat peanut butter
¼ cup sucralose-brown sugar blend
1 cup water

¾ cup egg substitute
¼ cup vegetable oil
⅓ cup mini semisweet chocolate chips
¼ cup peanut butter chips
¼ cup roasted peanuts, finely chopped

1. Preheat oven to 350°F. Lightly spray 13×9-inch baking pan with nonstick cooking spray.

2. Beat cake mix, peanut butter and sucralose-brown sugar blend in large bowl with electric mixer at low speed until mixture resembles coarse crumbs. Remove ⅓ cup to medium bowl for topping. Add water, egg substitute and oil to remaining mixture; beat at medium speed until well blended.

3. Spread batter evenly in prepared pan. Add chocolate chips, peanut butter chips and peanuts to reserved crumb mixture; mix well. Sprinkle over batter.

4. Bake 38 to 42 minutes or until toothpick inserted into center comes out clean. Cool cake completely in pan on wire rack.

Makes 24 servings

Dietary Exchanges: 1½ Diabetic Carb Count, 1½ Bread/Starch, 1½ Fat

Calories 203, **Total Fat** 10g, **Saturated Fat** 2g, **Protein** 4g, **Carbohydrates** 25g, **Cholesterol** 0mg, **Dietary Fiber** 1g, **Sodium** 226mg

January 20

If you haven't had Brussels sprouts since you were a kid, take a chance on them again. If you've only eaten them boiled, try roasting or steaming them. They're a great source of fiber and vitamins C, A, and K.

December 26

It's easy to put off workouts at the end of the year, saying you'll start fresh in the New Year. Try to work out, though, even if you shorten your usual exercise time. Sometimes, just getting off the couch and starting the workout can motivate you to do more!

1 tablespoon vegetable oil
1 pound Brussels sprouts, ends trimmed
    and discarded, thinly sliced

¼ cup dried cranberries
2 teaspoons packed brown sugar
¼ teaspoon salt

1. Heat oil in large skillet over medium-high heat. Add Brussels sprouts; cook and stir 10 minutes or until crisp-tender and beginning to brown. Add cranberries, brown sugar and salt; cook and stir 5 minutes or until browned.

Makes 4 servings

Dietary Exchanges: ½ Fat, ½ Fruit, 2 Vegetable

Calories 105, **Total Fat** 4g, **Saturated Fat** 1g, **Protein** 3g, **Carbohydrates** 17g, **Cholesterol** 0mg, **Dietary Fiber** 4g, **Sodium** 317mg

December 25

Fill your day with happiness—with thoughts of people who have been there for you, with gratitude for the good things in your life, and with appreciation for the good things in store.

January 22

Get the most out of visits with your healthcare providers. If you have questions or concerns, jot them down before you go to your visit so you'll be sure to remember them while you're at the office or clinic.

½ cup (1 stick) unsalted butter, softened
½ (8-ounce) package light cream cheese, softened
½ cup sugar
1 egg
1 egg white

1 teaspoon almond extract
½ teaspoon vanilla
2 cups all-purpose flour
½ teaspoon salt
12 teaspoons fruit spread, any flavor

1. Preheat oven to 350°F. Line cookie sheets with parchment paper. Beat butter, cream cheese and sugar in large bowl with electric mixer until light and fluffy. Add egg, egg white, almond and vanilla extracts; beat until well blended. Add flour and salt; beat until smooth and well blended.

2. Roll dough into 24 (1-inch) balls. Place on prepared cookie sheets. Using back of small spoon or thumb, make indentation in center of each ball; fill with ½ teaspoon fruit spread.

3. Bake 12 to 15 minutes until firm to touch and jam is bubbly. (Cookies will not brown.) Remove to wire racks; cool completely.

Makes 2 dozen cookies
Dietary Exchanges: 1 Bread/Starch, 1 Fat

Calories 111, **Total Fat** 5g, **Saturated Fat** 3g, **Protein** 2g, **Carbohydrates** 14g, **Cholesterol** 21mg, **Dietary Fiber** 0g, **Sodium** 76mg

January 23

Acronym Alert: CDE and RD

A certified diabetic educator (CDE) is a health professional who is trained to help people with diabetes manage the disease. CDEs are certified by the National Certification Board for Diabetes Educators.

An RD is a registered dietician. Some RDs specialize in diabetes education, and they can help you design a healthy meal plan.

December 23

Inspirations for research and treatment can come from strange places! The medication Exenatide (it's an injected drug) is a synthetic version of a hormone called extendin-4, which is found in the spit of the Gila monster. The desert lizard eats only a few times a year, and the hormone stimulates production in its pancreas, which is usually inactive.

2 to 3 carrots, shredded (1½ cups)
¼ cup raisins
¼ cup canned crushed pineapple, drained

1 tablespoon plain fat-free yogurt
4 lettuce leaves (optional)

1. Combine carrots, raisins, pineapple and yogurt in large bowl.

2. Refrigerate 2 hours and stir occasionally. Serve on lettuce leaves, if desired.

Makes 4 servings (½ cup per serving)

Dietary Exchanges: 1 Fruit

Calories 60, **Total Fat** 0g, **Saturated Fat** 0g, **Protein** 1g, **Carbohydrates** 14g, **Cholesterol** 0mg, **Dietary Fiber** 2g, **Sodium** 30mg

December 22

If you have problems with frequent heartburn, here are some steps you can take:

• Check the list of side effects for any medications you are taking. Some oral drugs for diabetes can cause gastrointestinal issues.

• Elevate the top half of your body when you sleep, to keep stomach acids in the stomach.

• Avoid spicy and acidic foods. Some people also have problems with chocolate and peppermint.

January 25

Cutting Down on Salt

While some sodium is necessary, most people have too much sodium in their diet. That contributes to high blood pressure, which is common in people with type 2 diabetes. High blood pressure increases the risk of heart attack, stroke, and kidney problems. Keep an eye on food labels to see how much sodium you're taking in—the American Heart Association recommends limiting sodium intake to 1,500 mg a day. Buy low-sodium options of foods like soup, soy sauce, and teriyaki sauce.

1 cup prepared mashed potatoes
½ cup finely chopped broccoli or spinach
2 egg whites

4 tablespoons shredded Parmesan cheese, divided

1. Preheat oven to 400°F. Spray 18 mini (1¾-inch) muffin cups with nonstick cooking spray.

2. Combine mashed potatoes, broccoli, egg whites and 2 tablespoons cheese in large bowl; mix well. Spoon evenly into prepared muffin cups. Top evenly with remaining 2 tablespoons cheese.

3. Bake 20 to 23 minutes or until golden brown. To remove from pan, gently run knife around outer edges and lift out with fork. Serve warm.

Makes 18 puffs (about 6 servings)

Dietary Exchanges: ½ Fat, 1 Vegetable

Calories 63, **Total Fat** 2g, **Saturated Fat** 1g, **Protein** 32g, **Carbohydrates** 8g, **Cholesterol** 2mg, **Dietary Fiber** 1g, **Sodium** 99mg

January 26

In addition to cutting down on salt, you can also help your blood pressure by adding certain foods into your diet. Look for foods rich in magnesium (nuts, seeds, dried beans), potassium (bananas, leafy greens, other fruits and vegetables), and calcium (dairy products).

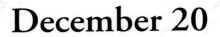

December 20

As the days get shorter and the weather gets colder, keep an eye on your mental health. Make sure that you're keeping up routines and staying connected with family and friends.

January 27

Myth or Fact? Fat and protein do not affect your blood glucose levels. Only carbohydrates do that.

Myth. Any food that contains calories will make your blood glucose levels rise. However, carbohydrates have the greatest direct effect.

December 19

If you're craving treats that a colleague has brought into the office, try a few of these strategies:

• Ask yourself if you're really hungry or if you're just eating because the food is there. Take a quick walk when you take a break instead of heading to a food table.

• Ask your colleague to move the treats across the desk or to a different location, so they're not directly in your line of sight.

• Don't always deny yourself—plan ahead for a small treat!

3 (6- to 7-inch) flour tortillas
Nonstick cooking spray
1 tablespoon sugar
⅛ teaspoon ground cinnamon
Dash ground allspice
1 container (6 ounces) nonfat
vanilla yogurt

1 teaspoon grated orange peel
1½ cups fresh strawberries,
stemmed and cut into quarters
½ cup fresh blueberries
4 teaspoons mini semisweet
chocolate chips

1. Preheat oven to 375°F. Cut each tortilla into 8 wedges. Place on ungreased baking sheet. Generously spray tortilla wedges with cooking spray. Combine sugar, cinnamon and allspice in small bowl. Sprinkle over tortilla wedges. Bake 7 to 9 minutes or until lightly browned; cool completely.

2. Meanwhile, combine yogurt and orange peel in small bowl.

3. Place 6 tortilla wedges on each of 4 small plates. Top with strawberries and blueberries. Drizzle with yogurt mixture; sprinkle with chocolate chips. Serve immediately.

Makes 4 servings

Dietary Exchanges: 1 Bread/Starch, ½ Fat, 1 Fruit

Calories 160, **Total Fat** 3g, **Saturated Fat** 1g, **Protein** 4g, **Carbohydrates** 28g, **Cholesterol** 2mg, **Dietary Fiber** 3g, **Sodium** 146mg

December 18

If you live in an area with snow, be aware that shoveling snow isn't just a chore, but an intense physical activity. As with any outdoor winter activity, dress warmly, warm up with some stretches before you go outside, take breaks, watch for dehydration, and monitor your blood glucose levels. And if you have heart problems, talk to your doctor first—it's possible that shoveling isn't a safe activity for you.

January 29

Do you and your family, friends, and colleagues know the symptoms of hypoglycemia? Make sure they have the information they need to help you when you need it.*

People who take insulin are at greater risk for hypoglycemic reactions—if you take insulin, talk to your doctor about getting a glucagon emergency kit.

More information on hypoglycemia can be found in the final pages of this calendar.

¼ to ½ teaspoon dried thyme

⅛ teaspoon salt

⅛ teaspoon black pepper

2 boneless pork loin chops (3 ounces each), trimmed of fat

⅔ cup unsweetened apple juice

½ small apple, sliced

2 tablespoons sliced green onion

2 tablespoons dried tart cherries

1 teaspoon cornstarch

1 tablespoon water

1. Combine thyme, salt and pepper in small bowl. Rub onto both sides of pork chops.

2. Spray large skillet with cooking spray; heat over medium heat. Add pork chops; cook 3 to 5 minutes or until barely pink in center, turning once. Remove to plate; keep warm.

3. Add apple juice, apple slices, green onion and cherries to same skillet. Simmer 2 to 3 minutes or until apple and onion are tender.

4. Stir cornstarch into water in small bowl until smooth; stir into skillet. Bring to a boil; cook and stir until thickened. Spoon apple mixture over pork chops.

Makes 2 servings (1 pork chop with about ½ cup apple-cherry glaze)

Dietary Exchanges: 1 Fat, 1½ Fruit, 2 Meat

Calories 243, **Total Fat** 8g, **Saturated Fat** 3g, **Protein** 19g, **Carbohydrates** 23g, **Cholesterol** 40mg, **Dietary Fiber** 1g, **Sodium** 191mg

January 30

People who have had diabetes for a long time can develop something called hypoglycemia unawareness, where they don't recognize the symptoms of low blood sugar. If you've been diagnosed with hypoglycemia unawareness, plan ahead. Stash sugar everywhere, wear ID, and invest in a glucagon emergency kit.

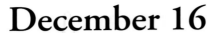

December 16

If you're sending out holiday cards, add a note of gratitude to any close friends who have gone above and beyond in helping you manage your diabetes!

⅓ cup dried apples
¼ cup dried apricots
¼ cup apple butter
2 tablespoons golden raisins
1 tablespoon reduced-fat peanut butter

½ cup reduced-fat granola
¼ cup graham cracker crumbs, divided
¼ cup mini chocolate chips
1 tablespoon water

1. Combine apples, apricots, apple butter, raisins and peanut butter in food processor or blender; process until smooth. Stir in granola, 1 tablespoon graham cracker crumbs, chocolate chips and water. Shape mixture into 16 balls.

2. Place remaining crumbs in shallow dish; roll balls in crumbs. Cover and refrigerate until ready to serve.

Makes 8 servings

Dietary Exchanges: 1 Bread/Starch, ½ Fat, ½ Fruit

Calories 121, **Total Fat** 4g, **Saturated Fat** 1g, **Protein** 3g, **Carbohydrates** 20g, **Cholesterol** 0mg, **Dietary Fiber** 2g, **Sodium** 14mg

December 15

Before modern, disposable needles became available, people with diabetes injected insulin with thick glass needles that had to be sterilized in boiling water every day and sharpened with a pumice stone or razor strap.

February 1

February is American Heart Month! What heart-healthy choices do you make in your daily life? If there are other steps you can take that you've been putting off, this month is a great time to put them into practice.

One resource for ideas and information is the web site of the American Heart Association (www.heart.org). Founded in 1924, the Association today has more than 22 million volunteers and supporters.

December 14

Quick Quiz

Most pancreas transplants are done:

A. In conjunction with liver transplants
B. In conjunction with kidney transplants
C. As a standalone procedure
D. In conjunction with spleen removal

Answer: B. The vast majority of pancreas transplants are performed
in conjunction with kidney transplants. Research shows that the
organs function better when they are both replaced.

February 2

Cardiovascular disease is the leading cause of death for Americans, and people with diabetes are at higher risk for heart disease. The good news is that bringing your blood sugar under control greatly reduces your risk for heart disease.

1 large acorn or golden acorn squash
¼ cup water
2 tablespoons pure maple syrup

1 tablespoon margarine or butter, melted
¼ teaspoon ground cinnamon

1. Preheat oven to 375°F.

2. Cut stem and blossom ends from squash. Cut squash crosswise into 4 equal slices. Discard seeds and membrane. Place water in 13×9-inch baking dish. Arrange squash in dish; cover with foil. Bake 30 minutes or until tender.

3. Combine maple syrup, margarine and cinnamon in small bowl; mix well. Uncover squash; pour off water. Brush squash with syrup mixture, letting excess pool in center of squash rings.

4. Bake 10 minutes or until syrup mixture is bubbly.

Makes 4 or 5 servings

Dietary Exchanges: 1 Bread/Starch, ½ Fat

Calories 90, **Total Fat** 3g, **Saturated Fat** 0.5g, **Protein** 1g, **Carbohydrates** 18g, **Cholesterol** 8mg, **Dietary Fiber** 2g, **Sodium** 39mg

4 teaspoons trans-fat-free margarine, divided

4 slices reduced-calorie whole wheat bread, toasted

3 ounces 96% fat-free diced ham

1 cup cholesterol-free egg substitute

¼ cup (1 ounce) reduced-fat sharp Cheddar cheese, grated

¼ teaspoon black pepper

⅛ teaspoon salt (optional)

1. Spread 1 teaspoon margarine on each bread slice and cut into ½-inch cubes.

2. Meanwhile, heat large skillet coated with nonstick cooking spray over medium heat. Add ham and cook 3 minutes or until beginning to lightly brown, stirring occasionally. Add egg substitute, tilt skillet to coat bottom and stir occasionally until almost set. Fold in toast cubes, cheese, pepper and salt, if desired.

3. Spoon equal amounts into 4 cups, bowls or travel mugs

Makes 4 servings (1 cup per serving)

Dietary Exchanges: ½ Bread/Starch, 2 Meat

Calories 130, **Total Fat** 4g, **Saturated Fat** 2g, **Protein** 13g, **Carbohydrates** 12g, **Cholesterol** 16mg, **Dietary Fiber** 3g, **Sodium** 550mg

December 12

Legendary hockey player Bobby Clarke, who helped lead the Philadelphia Flyers to two Stanley Cup victories, played with diabetes throughout his professional career, after being diagnosed with type 1 as an adolescent. Clarke was inducted into the Hockey Hall of Fame in 1987.

February 4

It's easy to fall into winter doldrums and let your activity levels drop. Here are a few ways you can counter that trend:

• Schedule a standing workout date with a friend. It's easy to let a trip to the gym slide, but harder to cancel on a workout buddy.

• Instead of sitting at your desk while you're on the phone, stand and walk around.

• Instead of going to the movies, go bowling.

December 11

Protect your feet from the cold! Wear warm socks or fleece-lined boots in cold temperatures. Wear socks at night. Don't use heating pads or hot water bottles to warm your feet, though, as they may cause burns.

February 5

One early, detailed description of diabetes comes from the Greek physician Aretaeus, who lived in the region of Cappadocia in what is now Turkey in the first century A.D. He also described tetanus, pneumonia, asthma, and epilepsy.

December 10

Stress-buster

If you know you have a busy month coming up, book some downtime into your schedule—a massage, some time with a valued friend, a few hours at a café with a book.

Pizza-Stuffed Potatoes

4 medium potatoes
   (about 7 ounces each)
¾ cup pizza sauce
⅛ teaspoon garlic powder
2 teaspoons grated Parmesan cheese

1 ounce turkey pepperoni slices
   (about 16), quartered
¾ cup shredded part-skim
   mozzarella cheese

1. Poke potatoes with fork and heat in microwave on HIGH 5 to 7 minutes or until soft. Split potatoes open with a knife; mash insides lightly.

2. Top each potato with 3 tablespoons pizza sauce and mix lightly into potato.

3. Sprinkle potatoes evenly with garlic powder and Parmesan cheese. Top evenly with pepperoni and mozzarella cheese.

4. Return potatoes to microwave and cook on HIGH 1 minute or until cheese is melted.

Makes 4 servings (1 potato per serving)

Dietary Exchanges: 3 Bread/Starch, 1 Meat

Calories 258, **Total Fat** 5g, **Saturated Fat** 2g, **Protein** 13g, **Carbohydrates** 42g, **Cholesterol** 23mg, **Dietary Fiber** 5g, **Sodium** 547mg

1 cup uncooked quinoa

2 cups water

2 tablespoons finely grated orange peel, plus additional for garnish

¼ cup fresh orange juice

2 teaspoons olive oil

½ teaspoon salt

¼ teaspoon ground cinnamon

⅓ cup dried cranberries

⅓ cup toasted pistachio nuts

1. Place quinoa in fine-mesh strainer; rinse well under cold running water. Bring 2 cups water to a boil in small saucepan; stir in quinoa. Reduce heat to low; cover and simmer 10 to 15 minutes or until quinoa is tender and water is absorbed. Stir in 2 tablespoons orange peel.

2. Whisk orange juice, oil, salt and cinnamon in small bowl. Pour over quinoa; gently toss to coat. Fold in cranberries and pistachios. Serve warm or at room temperature. Garnish with additional orange peel.

Makes 6 servings

Dietary Exchanges: 2 Bread/Starch, 1 Fat

Calories 185, **Total Fat** 6g, **Saturated Fat** 1g, **Protein** 5g, **Carbohydrates** 27g, **Cholesterol** 0mg, **Dietary Fiber** 3g, **Sodium** 198mg

February 7

Myth or Fact? All women who have gestational diabetes during a pregnancy will develop type 2 diabetes later in life.

Myth. However, women who have gestational diabetes do stand a 20 to 50 percent risk of developing type 2 diabetes within a decade. They are also more likely to develop gestational diabetes during a later pregnancy.

December 8

SEASONAL FOOD SPOTLIGHT

Cranberries are low in fat and high in fiber. They also contain vitamin C and manganese. Cranberries have anti-inflammatory benefits and cardiovascular benefits as well. If you're eating or drinking cranberry products, though, check the sugar content.

February 8

Cutting Down on Salt

One way to cut down on salt is to buy fresh. Fresh poultry, fish, and lean meats contain much less sodium than canned, smoked, and processed meats. When you do buy canned foods, such as canned tuna, rinse the meat to remove some of the sodium.

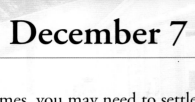

December 7

Sometimes, you may need to settle for less-than-optimal control on days your schedule is off. Do the best you can, but don't give up on activities you enjoy.

February 9

Acronym Alert: BMI

BMI stands for Body Mass Index. It's a tool to determine whether your weight is proportionate to your height. To calculate your BMI, multiply your weight in pounds by 700. Then divide the result by your height in inches. Then divide that result by your height in inches again. For instance, if your weight is 150 pounds and your height is 5'4", or 64", you would first multiply 150 by 700. Then you would divide the result, 105,000, by 64. Then you would divide the result by 64 again. The resulting BMI is 25.7.

Your goal is to have a BMI between 18.5 and 24.9. A BMI of 30 or over indicates obesity.

½ pound 95% lean ground beef
⅓ cup chopped onion
1 clove garlic, minced
1 can (8 ounces) tomato sauce
⅓ cup chopped carrot

¼ cup water
2 tablespoons red wine
1 teaspoon Italian seasoning
1½ cups hot cooked penne pasta
Chopped fresh parsley

1. Brown beef, onion and garlic in medium saucepan over medium-high heat 6 to 8 minutes, stirring to break up meat. Drain fat.

2. Add tomato sauce, carrot, water, wine and Italian seasoning; bring to a boil. Reduce heat; simmer 15 minutes.

3. Serve sauce over pasta. Sprinkle with parsley.

Makes 2 servings

Dietary Exchanges: 2 Bread/Starch, 1 Vegetable, 2 Meat

Calories 292, **Total Fat** 5g, **Saturated Fat** 2g, **Protein** 21g, **Carbohydrates** 40g, **Cholesterol** 45mg, **Dietary Fiber** 4g, **Sodium** 734mg

1 package (10 ounces) ready-made whole wheat pizza crust

¼ cup peanut sauce

⅓ cup chopped cilantro

1¼ cups (4 ounces) shredded cooked chicken

½ cup diced cucumber

¾ cup fresh or canned bean sprouts, rinsed and drained

¾ cup shredded or matchstick carrots

⅓ cup sliced green onion

Chopped fresh cilantro (optional)

1. Preheat oven to 450°F. Place pizza crust on baking sheet. Spread peanut sauce in thin layer over crust within ½-inch of edge. Sprinkle with cilantro. Arrange chicken evenly over crust. Bake 8 minutes or until warm.

2. Sprinkle cucumber, bean sprouts, carrots and green onion over top of pizza. Cut into wedges and top with cilantro, if desired.

Makes 6 servings

Dietary Exchanges: 2 Bread/Starch, 1 Meat

Calories 220, **Total Fat** 5g, **Saturated Fat** 2g, **Protein** 15g, **Carbohydrates** 30g, **Cholesterol** 22mg, **Dietary Fiber** 6g, **Sodium** 418mg

December 5

Participating in special events with friends and family while taking care of diabetes can be tricky, but it's not impossible! The key is to plan ahead. You may want to ask your host what foods will be served and when food will be served—and carry crackers or juice just in case plans change unexpectedly.

February 11

Stress-buster

If you're often feeling overwhelmed and anxious, or if you're going through a particularly difficult time, consider seeing a therapist or counselor for a few sessions. Many people have found a form of counseling known as cognitive-behavioral therapy (CBT) to be useful—CBT helps a therapist identify and replace negative and destructive thoughts and behaviors with more positive alternatives.

December 4

Cutting Down on Salt

When eating those salty foods that you love, such as foods that are pickled, cured, or contain broth, serve yourself a set, small portion.

February 12

SEASONAL FOOD SPOTLIGHT

Jerusalem artichokes aren't actually artichokes (they don't come from Jerusalem, either). Also called sunchokes, these root vegetables are members of the sunflower family. They contain little fat, and they're chock full of fiber, potassium, and iron.

You can use them in much the same way you would use potatoes. One simple way to prepare them is to roast them with olive oil and herbs.

5 cups whole grain bread cubes
2 cups cooked broccoli, coarsely chopped
1 cup cooked mushrooms, chopped
½ cup sliced green onions
1¼ cups shredded Swiss cheese, divided

2 cups cholesterol-free egg substitute
2 cups fat-free (skim) milk
1 tablespoon Dijon mustard
½ teaspoon black pepper
¼ teaspoon salt

1. Layer bread, broccoli, mushrooms and green onions in greased 13×9 baking dish. Sprinkle ¾ cup cheese evenly over vegetables.

2. Whisk egg substitute, milk, mustard, pepper and salt in medium bowl. Pour over strata. Refrigerate, covered, overnight.

3. Preheat oven to 350°F. Bake, uncovered, 30 minutes.

4. Sprinkle remaining ½ cup cheese evenly over top. Bake 10 to 12 minutes or until knife inserted in center comes out clean. Let stand 10 minutes before cutting and serving.

Makes 8 to 12 servings

Dietary Exchanges: 1 Bread/Starch, 1 Fat, ½ Vegetable, 2 Meat

Calories 190, **Total Fat** 6g, **Saturated Fat** 3g, **Protein** 17g, **Carbohydrates** 18g, **Cholesterol** 15mg, **Dietary Fiber** 2g, **Sodium** 340mg

3 medium baking potatoes
(8 ounces each), peeled
1 tablespoon olive oil
⅛ teaspoon salt
⅛ teaspoon black pepper
¼ cup shredded Parmesan cheese

½ cup fat-free mayonnaise
1 teaspoon chopped fresh rosemary
or ½ teaspoon dried rosemary
½ teaspoon grated lemon peel
1 clove garlic, crushed

1. Preheat oven to 425°F. Cut each potato into 12 wedges. In medium bowl, toss potatoes with oil, salt and pepper. Place in single layer on baking sheet. Bake 20 minutes; turn. Bake an additional 10 minutes. Push potatoes together on baking sheet. Sprinkle cheese over potatoes. Bake an additional 5 minutes or until cheese is melted and potatoes are tender.

2. Meanwhile, stir together mayonnaise, rosemary, lemon peel and garlic. Serve as dipping sauce with potatoes.

Makes 4 servings (about 9 fries and 2 tablespoons sauce per serving)

Dietary Exchanges: 2 Bread/Starch, 1 Fat

Calories 184, **Total Fat** 6g, **Saturated Fat** 2g, **Carbohydrates** 30g, **Cholesterol** 8mg, **Dietary Fiber** 2g, **Sodium** 395mg

December 2

Myth or Fact? People who take insulin should inject it in the same location for consistency's sake.

Myth. People who take insulin should vary their injection sites so that lumps of fat don't build up at a specific place. People may also vary injection sites to affect how quickly the insulin will enter the bloodstream—the belly absorbs insulin more quickly than the outer thighs, for example.

February 14

Being diabetic doesn't mean giving up chocolate! In fact, chocolate contains antioxidants that provide good health benefits. Just keep your portions small, account for the effect it will have on your blood sugar, and where possible, opt for dark chocolate with a high cocoa content.

December 1

The first blood glucose meter was developed by the Ames Company in the 1970s. Before blood glucose meters were available, people with diabetes tested urine, not blood, when they needed to measure their blood sugar level.

February 15

NFL quarterback Jay Cutler was diagnosed with type 1 diabetes in 2008. His organization, the Jay Cutler Foundation, works to raise awareness of diabetes and helps send kids with diabetes to summer camp.

November 30

Sometimes when you're overwhelmed or stressed out, doing something small for yourself can put you in a better frame of mind. Buy a bunch of bright flowers, or pick up a loaf of fresh bread from the bakery.

February 16

Quick Quiz

Which of the following foods are good sources of omega 3 fatty acids, which tend to lower blood cholesterol and heart disease risk?

    A. Mackerel
    B. Canola oil
    C. Walnuts
    D. Flax seeds
    E. All of the above

Answer: E. All of the above.

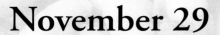

November 29

If you're drinking alcohol, always drink with a meal or shortly after eating, and check your blood sugar before the first sip.

2 large bunches kale (about 2 pounds)
2 tablespoons light butter-and-oil spread
2 tablespoons all-purpose flour
1½ cups fat-free (skim) milk
½ cup shredded Parmesan cheese, plus
   additional for garnish

2 cloves garlic, minced
¼ teaspoon salt
⅛ teaspoon ground nutmeg

1. Remove stems from kale; discard. Roughly chop leaves. Bring large saucepan of water to a boil. Add kale; cook 5 minutes. Drain.

2. Melt butter in large saucepan over medium heat. Stir in flour. Cook and stir 1 to 2 minutes or until smooth. Gradually whisk in milk until well blended. Whisk constantly over medium heat 4 to 5 minutes or until sauce boils and is thickened, scraping up browned bits occasionally. Whisk in ½ cup cheese, garlic, salt and nutmeg.

3. Remove saucepan from heat. Fold in kale until combined. Sprinkle with additional cheese, if desired.

Makes 8 servings

Dietary Exchanges: ½ Fat, 2 Vegetable

Calories 90, **Total Fat** 3g, **Saturated Fat** 1g, **Protein** 7g, **Carbohydrates** 10g, **Cholesterol** 5mg, **Dietary Fiber** 1g, **Sodium** 222mg

November 28

Quick Quiz

How much beer is considered a "drink"?

A. 2 ounces of beer
B. 8 ounces of beer
C. 12 ounces of beer
D. 18 ounces of beer

Answer: C. A "drink" usually means 12 ounces of beer, 5 ounces of wine, or 1.5 ounces of liquor. Drinking in moderation means no more than one drink for women or two for men per day.

February 18

One tip for eating healthy: Keep your plate colorful! The same chemicals that give some fruits and vegetables their bright rainbow of colors may also promote health and fight disease. For instance, greens such as kale, spinach, collards, and broccoli contain antioxidants that keep your eyes healthy.

November 27

The end of the year can be challenging for many people because of family gatherings and worsening weather that can disrupt food and exercise routines. Set a time each week for checking in on how you're doing in meeting your goals and strategizing for the coming week.

February 19

Being physical doesn't just help your body. When you exercise, your body produces chemical messengers called endorphins. Endorphins help relieve anxiety and pain.

November 26

Take a moment during the season of Thanksgiving to be thankful to those researchers and scientists who studied diabetes in order to make it more manageable. And think back on your own efforts and successes and be grateful for them!

¾ pound chicken tenders
Nonstick cooking spray
4 cups shredded stemmed spinach
2 cups washed and torn romaine lettuce
1 large grapefruit, peeled and sectioned
8 thin slices red onion, separated into rings

2 tablespoons (½ ounce) crumbled blue cheese
½ cup frozen citrus blend concentrate, thawed
¼ cup prepared fat-free Italian salad dressing

1. Cut chicken into 2×½-inch strips. Spray large nonstick skillet with cooking spray; heat over medium heat. Add chicken; cook and stir 5 minutes or until no longer pink in center. Remove from skillet.

2. Divide spinach, lettuce, grapefruit, onion, cheese and chicken among 4 salad plates. Combine citrus blend concentrate and Italian dressing in small bowl; drizzle over salads.

Makes 4 servings

Dietary Exchanges: 1 Fruit, 2 Vegetable, 2½ Meat

Calories 218, **Total Fat** 4g, **Saturated Fat** 1g, **Protein** 23g, **Carbohydrates** 23g, **Cholesterol** 55mg, **Dietary Fiber** 3g, **Sodium** 361mg

1 tablespoon olive oil
1 clove garlic, finely minced
1 tablespoon light butter-and-oil
   spread, melted

12 cups plain popped popcorn
⅓ cup finely grated Parmesan cheese
½ teaspoon dried basil
½ teaspoon dried oregano

1. Stir oil and garlic into spread in small bowl until well blended. Pour over popcorn in large bowl; toss to coat. Sprinkle with cheese, basil and oregano.

Makes 12 cups popcorn (about 6 servings)

Tip: One regular-size microwavable package of popcorn yields about 10 to 12 cups of popped popcorn.

Dietary Exchanges: 1 Bread/Starch, 1 Fat

Calories 110, **Total Fat** 5g, **Saturated Fat** 1g, **Protein** 4g, **Carbohydrates** 13g, **Cholesterol** 4mg, **Dietary Fiber** 2g, **Sodium** 83mg

February 21

One challenge that people with diabetes face is the reaction of others. People may have many questions. They may want to critique your eating habits or offer you advice (and sometimes, unfortunately, the advice may be based on misinformation). When you have the energy, it's great to take the opportunity to educate others! But don't be afraid to calmly, firmly redirect people to another topic. Your diabetes is not the most important thing about you.

November 24

The holiday season is a great time to let the people in our lives know that we're grateful for them. If there are members of your diabetic care team who have been especially helpful or kind, drop them a note or express your thanks in person at your next appointment!

February 22

Low in calories, cauliflower contains plenty of fiber, as well as vitamin C, vitamin K, vitamin B6, and iron. If you've only had it boiled or microwaved, try a different method of preparing it for variety. You can even mash cauliflower and season it with garlic like you would potatoes!

November 23

Don't limit your eating of turkey to the Thanksgiving season! Lean ground turkey can be used instead of ground beef in many recipes. Try turkey meatloaf, turkey tacos, or turkey burgers.

February 23

Some people feel that frequent blood glucose testing is an extra constraint on their time and energy. But in fact, once you begin to identify patterns in your blood glucose control based on diet, exercise, and medications, frequent testing can give you more freedom and less anxiety.

November 22

You may enjoy the fat-free or reduced fat versions of some foods. For other foods, you may find it better to cut down on the portion size, or substitute a different food altogether.

February 24

Here are five benefits to frequent testing of your blood glucose level.

- Reduced risk of long-term diabetes complications
- Quick identification and treatment of a low or high blood glucose level
- Ability to provide solid information to your health care providers so they can tailor your treatment plan
- Ability to evaluate whether your overall treatment plan is effective and whether any changes are working
- Increased control over the food you eat and the amount you exercise

November 21

We hear "no pain, no gain" when it comes to exercise, but that doesn't need to be true. Exercise with moderate intensity, doing activities you enjoy, and you'll be more likely to stick with them.

- 5 cups cauliflower florets (about 1¼ pounds)
- 1 tablespoon reduced-fat margarine, melted
- 1 small red bell pepper, cut into quarters
- 2 tablespoons water
- 3 large tomatoes, peeled, seeded and coarsely chopped
- 2 to 3 teaspoons chopped fresh tarragon
- ½ teaspoon chopped fresh parsley
- ⅓ cup (9 to 10) coarsely crushed unsalted saltine crackersd

1. Preheat oven to 450°F. Toss cauliflower with margarine in large bowl; place cauliflower and bell pepper, cut sides down, in single layer in shallow baking pan. Add water to pan. Bake 15 minutes. *Reduce oven temperature to 425°F.*

2. Bake 25 to 28 minutes or until cauliflower is tender and golden brown and bell pepper skin is blistered. Remove bell pepper pieces to plate and transfer cauliflower to 11×7-inch baking dish. *Reduce oven temperature to 400°F.*

3. Remove and discard skin from bell pepper. Place tomatoes and bell pepper in food processor; process until smooth. Add tarragon and parsley; process until blended. Pour tomato sauce over cauliflower.

4. Bake 10 minutes or until hot and bubbly. Sprinkle with cracker crumbs before serving.

Makes 5 servings

Dietary Exchanges: ½ Fat, 2½ Vegetable, **Calories** 80, **Total Fat** 2g, **Saturated Fat** 1g, **Protein** 3g, **Carbohydrates** 14g, **Cholesterol** 0mg, **Dietary Fiber** 4g, **Sodium** 100mg

2 packages (10 ounces each) frozen chopped broccoli

1 cup fat-free reduced-sodium chicken or vegetable broth

2 tablespoons reduced-fat mayonnaise

2 teaspoons dried minced onion (optional)

1. Combine broccoli, chicken broth, mayonnaise and onion, if desired, in large saucepan. Simmer, covered, stirring occasionally, until broccoli is tender.

2. Uncover; continue to simmer, stirring occasionally, until liquid has evaporated.

Makes 7 servings

Dietary Exchanges: 1 Vegetable

Calories 31, **Total Fat** 1g, **Saturated Fat** 1g, **Protein** 2g, **Carbohydrates** 4g, **Cholesterol** 1mg, **Dietary Fiber** 2g, **Sodium** 26mg

February 26

If you haven't exercised regularly in a while, ease back into it with low-impact aerobic exercises that don't put strain on your muscles, bones, and joints. Swimming, cycling, hiking, rowing, using an elliptical trainer, and dancing are all good examples of low-impact aerobic exercises. And talk to a doctor or exercise physiologist before you begin.

November 19

Broccoli and cauliflower are members of the *cruciferous* family, along with cabbage, bok choy, kale, and horseradish. When you're planning meals, pack in plenty of cruciferous vegetables. They tend to have lots of varied nutrients and health benefits.

February 27

Even if you work hard to control your blood sugar, diabetes is a progressive disease. At some point, you may need to adjust your medication or add insulin to your treatment. Don't give in to feelings of discouragement—use all the tools at your disposal!

November 18

Sometimes, well-intentioned friends may be persistent in suggesting foods, desserts, or eating strategies that don't fit into your meal plans. Don't be afraid to set boundaries, calmly and firmly, without getting bogged down in arguments and explanations.

Nonstick cooking spray
¼ cup chopped green or red bell pepper
2 tablespoons sliced green onion
1 slice (1 ounce) reduced-fat smoked deli ham, chopped
½ cup cholesterol-free egg substitute
Black pepper
4 slices multigrain or whole grain bread
2 slices (¾-ounce each) reduced-fat Cheddar or Swiss cheese

1. Spray small skillet with cooking spray; heat over medium heat. Add bell pepper and green onion; cook and stir 4 minutes or until crisp-tender. Stir in ham.

2. Whisk egg substitute and black pepper in small bowl until well blended. Pour egg mixture into skillet; cook 2 minutes or until egg mixture is almost set, stirring occasionally.

3. Heat grill pan or medium skillet over medium heat. Spray one side of each bread slice with cooking spray; turn bread over. Top each bread slice with 1 cheese slice and half of egg mixture. Top with second bread slice. Repeat with remaining bread slices, cheese slices and egg mixture.

4. Grill 2 minutes per side, pressing down lightly with spatula until toasted. (Cover pan with lid during last 2 minutes of cooking to melt cheese.) Serve immediately.

Makes 2 sandwiches

Dietary Exchanges: 2 Bread/Starch, 2 Meat, **Calories** 271, **Total Fat** 5g, **Saturated Fat** 1g, **Protein** 24g, **Carbohydrates** 30g, **Cholesterol** 9mg, **Dietary Fiber** 6g, **Sodium** 577mg

November 17

When Grammy-winning singer Patti LaBelle was diagnosed with type 2 diabetes in 1995, she responded by working to raise awareness of the disease. She even produced a cookbook with healthy, diabetic-friendly recipes, *Patti LaBelle's Lite Cuisine*.

February 29

Did you know that most people experience a spike in blood sugar in the morning hours between 4 A.M. and 8 A.M.? It even has a name: the "dawn phenomenon." Blood sugar dips naturally by afternoon.

November 16

Stress-buster

Many people leave their home in a rush each morning. Make your mornings less stressful by preparing as much as you can the night before. Pack lunch, select an outfit, and make sure anything you might need (phone, keys, wallet, umbrella) are gathered together, ready to go.

March 1

Try to make an effort to add a little extra movement into your daily routine. Instead of searching for the closest parking space at the store, park your car further away. If you work or live in a building with elevators, take the stairs sometimes. If a commercial comes on while you're watching television, stand and walk in place.

1 package (10 ounces) frozen asparagus cuts
1 teaspoon lemon juice
3 to 4 drops hot pepper sauce
¼ teaspoon salt (optional)

¼ teaspoon dried basil
⅛ teaspoon black pepper
2 teaspoons sunflower kernels
Lemon slices (optional)

1. Place asparagus and 2 tablespoons water in 1-quart microwavable casserole dish; cover. Microwave on HIGH 4½ to 5½ minutes or until asparagus is hot, stirring after half the cooking time to break apart. Drain. Cover; set aside.

2. Combine lemon juice, hot pepper sauce, salt, basil and pepper in small bowl. Pour mixture over asparagus; toss to coat. Sprinkle with sunflower kernels. Garnish with lemon slices, if desired.

Makes 4 servings

Dietary Exchanges: 1 Vegetable

Calories 29, **Total Fat** 1g, **Saturated Fat** 1g, **Protein** 2g, **Carbohydrates** 4g, **Cholesterol** 0mg, **Dietary Fiber** 1g, **Sodium** 4mg

1 cup old-fashioned oats
¾ cup fat-free (skim) milk
1 egg white
2 tablespoons packed brown
   sugar, divided

1½ teaspoons freshly grated
   ginger *or* ¾ teaspoon ground ginger
½ ripe pear, diced

1. Preheat oven to 350°F. Spray 2 (6-ounce) ramekins with nonstick cooking spray.

2. Combine oats, milk, egg white, 1 tablespoon brown sugar and ginger in medium bowl; mix well. Pour evenly into ramekins. Top evenly with pear slices; sprinkle with remaining 1 tablespoon brown sugar.

3. Bake 15 minutes. Serve warm.

Makes 2 servings

Dietary Exchanges: 3½ Bread/Starch

Calories 268, **Total Fat** 3g, **Saturated Fat** 1g, **Protein** 10g, **Carbohydrates** 52g, **Cholesterol** 2mg, **Dietary Fiber** 5g, **Sodium** 70mg

November 14

Today is World Diabetes Day! November 14 was selected as the date to commemorate the birthday of Frederick Banting, the Canadian Nobel Prize Winner whose team was the first to administer insulin as a treatment for diabetes. His colleagues included Charles Best, John MacLeod, and James Collip.

March 3

Sushruta, an Indian surgeon who lived around 600 B.C., prescribed exercise for his patients with diabetes. In ancient India, the diagnosis for diabetes involved ants—the insects were attracted to the sugar-filled urine of people with the disease.

November 13

Quick Quiz

High blood sugar can affect your mental performance.

A. True
B. False

Answer: True. As blood sugar goes up, so do the number of mental errors and the time it takes to perform basic tasks. Wide variations in blood-sugar level have also been shown to hinder intellectual function.

March 4

Myth or Fact? Humans are the only mammals to get diabetes.

Myth. Dogs, cats, mice, and other animals that have a pancreas can develop diabetes. Properly treated, a beloved pet with diabetes can live a full and healthy life.

November 12

Diabetes is sometimes called a "family disease" because it tends to affect everyone in a family, not just the person with diabetes. Although the lifestyle changes that diabetes demands can be positive for everyone, they can also be overwhelming. Making a conscious effort to balance necessary discussions about the disease with other topics and interests can help.

March 5

Cutting Down on Salt

Try substituting other seasonings and spices for salt. Buy fresh herbs and use them in cooking, in salsa and dips, and in salads. You could even grow your own herbs in windowsill gardens!

One caution: Don't buy sea salt thinking it has less sodium than regular table salt. It generally does not.

½ cups (3 ounces) uncooked wagon wheel or rotelle pasta

3 ounces 95% lean ground beef

2 tablespoons chopped onion

2 tablespoons chopped green bell pepper

1 clove garlic, minced

½ cup fat-free pasta sauce

Dash black pepper

2 tablespoons shredded Italian-style mozzarella and Parmesan cheese blend

Peperoncini (optional)

1. Preheat oven to 350°F. Cook pasta according to package directions, omitting salt. Drain; return pasta to saucepan.

2. Meanwhile, heat medium nonstick skillet over medium-high heat. Add beef, onion, bell pepper and garlic; cook and stir 3 to 4 minutes or until beef is no longer pink and vegetables are crisp-tender. Drain.

3. Add beef mixture, pasta sauce and black pepper to pasta in saucepan; mix well. Spoon mixture into 1-quart baking dish. Sprinkle with cheese.

4. Bake 15 minutes or until heated through. Serve with peperoncini, if desired.

Makes 2 servings

Dietary Exchanges: 2 Bread/Starch, 1 Fat, 2 Vegetable, 1 Meat

Calories 282, **Total Fat** 7g, **Saturated Fat** 3g, **Protein** 16g, **Carbohydrates** 37g, **Cholesterol** 31mg, **Dietary Fiber** 3g, **Sodium** 368mg

4 ounces uncooked multigrain rotini pasta

2 cups diced cooked chicken

½ cup chopped roasted red bell peppers

12 pitted kalamata olives, halved

1½ tablespoons olive oil

1 tablespoon dried basil

1 tablespoon cider vinegar

1 to 2 cloves garlic, minced

¼ teaspoon salt (optional

1. Cook pasta according to package directions, omitting salt. Drain well; cool.

2. Combine chicken, peppers, olives, oil, basil, vinegar, garlic and salt, if desired, in large bowl.

3. Add cooled pasta to chicken mixture; toss gently. Divide equally among 4 plates.

Makes 4 servings

Dietary Exchanges: 1½ Bread/Starch, 3 Meat

Calories 276, **Total Fat** 9g, **Saturated Fat** 2g, **Protein** 25g, **Carbohydrates** 25g, **Cholesterol** 54mg, **Dietary Fiber** 3g, **Sodium** 341mg

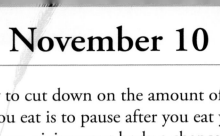

November 10

One way to cut down on the amount of dessert you eat is to pause after you eat your main course, giving your body a chance to feel full. Build in a break to wash dishes or take a family walk. Then see if you're still hungry.

March 7

Build a variety of activities that challenge
different body parts into your exercise routine.
Cross-training helps you develop well-rounded
fitness and prevents soreness from overuse of
the same muscles and joints.

November 9

If you're branching out to try new foods and new recipes, don't forget to visit your local library—they may have cookbooks you can check out and browse through to find recipe ideas.

March 8

Look forward, not backward. Every day is a new chance to make new choices in your diet, your exercise habits, and how closely you monitor your blood glucose. Every day is a chance to build new habits that will help you manage your diabetes.

November 8

If you're sleeping badly, check your blood sugar levels. Having elevated blood sugar during the night keeps you at a shallow sleep level. Diabetes also increases the risk of developing sleep apnea, a disorder in which the sleeper snores loudly and actually stops breathing multiple times per night.

March 9

Quick Quiz

Which statement about cholesterol is true?

A. All cholesterol is bad, but LDL is worse than HDL.
B. All cholesterol is bad, but HDL is worse than LDL.
C. HDL cholesterol removes fatty acids from your arteries, while LDL cholesterol deposits fat in the walls of your arteries.
D. LDL cholesterol removes fatty acids from your arteries, while HDL cholesterol deposits fat in the walls of your arteries.

Answer: C. HDL cholesterol is the "good" cholesterol that removes fatty acids from your arteries.

Nonstick cooking spray
4 (8-inch) flour tortillas
¾ cup (3 ounces) shredded reduced-fat
   Monterey Jack or Cheddar cheese
½ cup canned black beans, rinsed
   and drained

2 green onions, sliced
¼ cup chopped fresh cilantro
½ teaspoon ground cumin
½ cup salsa
2 tablespoons plus 2 teaspoons fat-free
   sour cream

1. Preheat oven to 450°F. Spray large nonstick baking sheet with nonstick cooking spray. Place 2 tortillas on prepared baking sheet; sprinkle each with half the cheese.

2. Combine beans, green onions, cilantro and cumin in small bowl; mix lightly. Spoon bean mixture evenly over cheese; top with remaining tortillas. Spray tops with cooking spray.

3. Bake 10 to 12 minutes or until cheese is melted and tortillas are lightly browned. Cut into quarters; top each tortilla wedge with 1 tablespoon salsa and 1 teaspoon sour cream.

Makes 8 servings

Dietary Exchanges: 1 Bread/Starch, ½ Meat

Calories 105, **Total Fat** 4g, **Saturated Fat** 1g, **Protein** 7g, **Carbohydrates** 13g, **Cholesterol** 8mg, **Dietary Fiber** 1g, **Sodium** 259mg

4 fresh or thawed frozen tilapia fillets about ¾ inch thick and 4 ounces each)

Black pepper

½ cup fat-free sour cream

2 tablespoons chopped fresh dill

4 teaspoons Dijon mustard

2 teaspoons lemon juice

⅛ teaspoon garlic powder

1. Preheat broiler. Lightly spray rack of broiler pan with nonstick cooking spray. Place fish on rack. Sprinkle with pepper. Broil 4 to 5 inches from heat 5 to 8 minutes or until fish begins to flake when tested with fork. (It is not necessary to turn fish.)

2. Meanwhile, combine sour cream, dill, mustard, lemon juice and garlic powder in small bowl. Serve over warm fish.

Makes 4 servings

Dietary Exchanges: 3 Meat

Calories 142, **Total Fat** 3g, **Saturated Fat** 0g, **Protein** 22g, **Carbohydrates** 8g, **Cholesterol** 5mg, **Dietary Fiber** 1g, **Sodium** 200mg

November 6

If you live in an area that gets a lot of
rain, snow, or cold in the fall and winter,
plan ahead for indoor exercise. Search
out enjoyable activities that get you up
and moving: architectural tours of local
buildings, food drives, or classes in sculpting
or making stained glass.

March 11

Healthy eating starts at the planning and shopping stages. When you're looking over recipes, look at the nutritional information. Can you substitute alternate ingredients for salt or full-fat ingredients? When you're shopping, pay attention to how much time you spent on the outskirts of the store (where most of the fresh foods are stocked) versus the interior aisles where you find pre-packaged foods that are often less healthy.

November 5

People with type 1 diabetes can develop type 2 diabetes later in life. People with type 2 are very unlikely to develop type 1, though.

March 12

When you're making changes in how you eat or exercise, implement them gradually. Many people have had the experience of falling away from a strict diet full of bland or tasteless foods and quickly gaining back the weight they lost. Instead, move to eating healthy foods that you enjoy, for long-lasting, sustainable change.

November 4

Cutting Down on Salt

Buy unsalted butter (1 tbsp has only 2 mg of sodium) rather than salted butter, especially for baking. When you're eating bread, dip it in flavored olive oil instead of slathering on the butter.

Keep an eye on expiration dates; unsalted butter does not last as long as salted butter.

1½ teaspoons fresh rosemary leaves, minced, *or* ½ teaspoon dried rosemary

2 cloves garlic, minced

¾ teaspoon black pepper

½ teaspoon salt

6 boneless skinless chicken breasts (about ¼ pound each)

1 tablespoon olive oil

¼ cup balsamic vinegar

1. Combine rosemary, garlic, pepper and salt in small bowl; mix well. Place chicken in large bowl; drizzle chicken with oil and rub with spice mixture. Cover and refrigerate several hours.

2. Preheat oven to 450°F. Spray heavy roasting pan or cast iron skillet with nonstick cooking spray. Place chicken in pan; bake 10 minutes. Turn chicken over, stirring in 3 to 4 tablespoons water if drippings begin to stick to pan.

3. Bake about 10 minutes or until chicken is golden brown and no longer pink in center. If pan is dry, stir in another 1 to 2 tablespoons water to loosen drippings.

4. Drizzle vinegar over chicken in pan. Transfer chicken to plates. Stir liquid in pan; drizzle over chicken. Garnish, if desired.

Makes 6 servings

Dietary Exchanges: 3 Meat

Calories 174, **Total Fat** 5g, **Saturated Fat** 1g, **Protein** 27g, **Carbohydrates** 3g, **Cholesterol** 73mg, **Dietary Fiber** 1g, **Sodium** 242mg

1 package (11 ounces) refrigerated
    breadstick dough
2 tablespoons apple butter

1 to 1½ teaspoons orange juice
¼ cup sifted powdered sugar
⁄ teaspoon grated orange peel (optional)

1. Preheat oven to 350°F. Spray baking sheet with nonstick cooking spray; set aside.

2. Unroll breadstick dough. Separate along perforations into 12 pieces. Gently stretch each piece to 9 inches in length. Twist ends of each piece in opposite directions 3 to 4 times. Coil each twisted strip into snail shape on prepared baking sheet. Tuck ends underneath.

3. Use thumb to make small indentation in center of each breadstick coil. Spoon about ½ teaspoon apple butter into each indentation. Bake 11 to 13 minutes or until golden brown. Remove from baking sheet. Cool on wire rack 10 minutes.

4. Meanwhile, stir enough orange juice into powdered sugar in small bowl to make a pourable glaze. Stir in orange peel, if desired. Drizzle over rolls. Serve warm.

Makes 12 servings

Dietary Exchanges: 1½ Bread/Starch

Calories 105, **Total Fat** 1g, **Saturated Fat** 1g, **Protein** 2g, **Carbohydrates** 21g, **Cholesterol** 0mg, **Dietary Fiber** 1g, **Sodium** 186mg

March 14

Stress-buster

Instead of getting impatient or angry when you are stuck in a long line or have to wait at a doctor's office, plan ahead. Bring along a tablet loaded with games, a small puzzle booklet, or a magazine you've wanted to read.

November 2

Myth or Fact? You can take a blood sample from any part of your body for glucose testing and get the same results.

Myth. Alternative site testing is possible with some meters, but blood sugar changes show up sooner in your fingertips than in other parts of your body—if you suspect your blood sugar is rising or falling quickly, use your fingertips.

March 15

Supreme Court Justice Sonia Sotomayor was diagnosed with type 1 diabetes when she was a young child. She's spoken candidly in interviews and her memoir about controlling her blood sugar and taking insulin.

November 1

In the United States, November is National Diabetes Month. That makes it a good time to visit the web site of the American Diabetes Association (http://diabetes.org/). Founded in 1940, the Association has developed a lot of good resources and educational material during its long history.

Point family and friends towards the diabetes risk test found there.

http://www.diabetes.org/are-you-at-risk/diabetes-risk-test/

March 16

Artichokes begin to come into season in the spring! Full of fiber, artichokes also provide vitamin C, vitamin K, and manganese.

October 31

Stock up on plenty of delicious snacks that are good for you—it'll help you resist the temptation to overindulge in Halloween candy.

1 tablespoon butter
2 small carrots, diagonally cut into thin slices
1 clove garlic, minced
½ teaspoon dried basil, dill weed or tarragon
1 small red bell pepper, cut into thin strips

1 medium yellow squash, cut into matchsticks
4 jarred artichoke hearts, drained and rinsed, cut into quarters
1½ teaspoons lemon juice
Salt and pepper

1. Melt butter in large skillet over medium heat. Add carrots, garlic and basil; cook and stir 2 minutes. Add bell pepper; cook and stir 2 minutes. Add yellow squash and artichokes; cook and stir 3 minutes.

2. Add lemon juice; cook and stir 1 minute. Season with salt and pepper.

Makes 2 servings

Dietary Exchanges: 1 Fat, 4 Vegetable

Calories 147, **Total Fat** 6g, **Saturated Fat** 3g, **Protein** 4g, **Carbohydrates** 22g, **Cholesterol** 15mg, **Dietary Fiber** 6g, **Sodium** 111mg

3 medium beets (red and/or golden), trimmed
1½ tablespoons extra virgin olive oil

¼ teaspoon salt
¼ teaspoon black pepper

1. Preheat oven to 300°F.

2. Cut beets into very thin slices, about ¹⁄₁₆ inch thick. Combine beets, oil, salt and pepper in medium bowl; gently toss to coat. Arrange in single layer on baking sheets.

3. Bake 30 to 35 minutes or until darkened and crisp.* Spread on paper towels to cool completely.

*If the beet chips are darkened but not crisp, turn oven off and let chips stand in oven until crisp, about 10 minutes. Do not keep the oven on as the chips will burn easily.

Makes 2 to 3 servings

Dietary Exchanges: 2 Fat, 2 Vegetable

Calories 144, **Total Fat** 10g, **Saturated Fat** 2g, **Protein** 2g, **Carbohydrates** 12g, **Cholesterol** 0mg, **Dietary Fiber** 4g, **Sodium** 386mg

March 18

Sometimes we don't see the immediate benefits of exercise—but exercise definitely pays over the long-term. Researchers at the Cooper Institute in Dallas, Texas, rated the activity level of more than 1,200 men with type 2 diabetes. A dozen years later, they showed that men who were physically active on a regular basis and were moderately fit had a 60 percent lower death rate than unfit men who didn't exercise.

October 29

Beets contain betalains, nutrients that have anti-oxidant properties. Betaleins are lost during the cooking process, so take care not to overcook your beets

March 19

If you find yourself stopping by the vending machines at work or school, pack a healthier snack to bring with you instead. Make sure it's something you honestly enjoy, so you won't be tempted to set it aside.

October 28

Get in a little extra activity: Take a walk around your neighborhood, or a nearby one, to see the Halloween decorations and the changing leaves.

March 20

When you're planning meals and snacks, don't forget to account for what you drink! If you're a fan of soda, reach for the diet—a serving of regular soda can contain as much as 40 grams of carbohydrate.

October 27

It's the season of pumpkin pie, but did you know that pumpkin seeds are a delicious, healthy snack? They offer zinc, magnesium, and vitamin E. As with most seeds and nuts, it's easy to overindulge, so measure out a portion rather than eating from the bag.

3 cups cubed (about ½ inch) peeled Yukon
  Gold potatoes (1 pound total)
1 tablespoon unsalted butter
⅔ cup diced onion
½ cup fat-free (skim) milk, warmed

2 tablespoons finely chopped
  fresh cilantro
½ teaspoon salt
¼ teaspoon black pepper

1. Place potatoes in large saucepan; cover with water. Cover; bring to a boil. Reduce heat; boil 15 minutes or until potatoes are tender when pierced with fork.

2. Meanwhile, melt butter in medium nonstick skillet over medium heat. Add onion; cook and stir 7 minutes or until browned.

3. Drain potatoes; return to pan. Reduce heat to very low. Stir in milk, onion, cilantro, salt and pepper. Mash with potato masher until smooth and well combined..

Makes 4 servings (about ½ cup per serving)

Dietary Exchanges: 2 Bread/Starch, ½ Fat

Calories 148, **Total Fat** 3g, **Saturated Fat** 2g, **Carbohydrates** 28g, **Cholesterol** 8mg, **Dietary Fiber** 3g, **Sodium** 311mg

1½ cups whole wheat blend pancake and waffle mix
½ cup plain nonfat Greek yogurt
½ cup fat-free (skim) milk
⅓ cup sugar

⅓ cup natural creamy peanut butter
1 egg
1 tablespoon vegetable oil
½ cup mini semisweet chocolate chips

1. Preheat oven to 350°F. Spray 9-inch square baking pan with nonstick cooking spray.

2. Beat pancake mix, yogurt, milk, sugar, peanut butter, egg and oil in large bowl with electric mixer at medium speed until smooth and well blended. Fold in chocolate chips. Pour into prepared pan.

3. Bake 25 minutes or until toothpick inserted into center comes out clean. Cool completely in pan on wire rack.

Makes 9 servings

Dietary Exchanges: 2 Bread/Starch, 2 Fat

Calories 245, **Total Fat** 9g, **Saturated Fat** 3g, **Protein** 8g, **Carbohydrates** 36g, **Cholesterol** 22mg, **Dietary Fiber** 3g, **Sodium** 467mg

March 22

According to the *National Diabetes Statistics Report*, about one quarter of people who have diabetes aren't diagnosed with it. Do the people in your life have information about diabetes, its symptoms, and its effects? A diagnosis gives people an opportunity to assemble a care team, take necessary medications or insulin, and enact lifestyle changes in order to prevent long-term damage.

October 25

There are treatments for those who suffer from pain from nerve damage. One treatment is capsaicin, a skin cream that contains the substance that puts the fire in cayenne peppers. The cream stings at first, but after repeated use, it appears to desensitize pain receptors.

March 23

Whole-grain breads, pasta, and rice tend to have more vitamins, fiber, and minerals than white bread, pasta, and rice. White rice and pasta go through a process called refining that strips out some of the nutrients. (To make things more complex, some nutrients are then put back through a process called enrichment.)

Many people who begin to eat whole-grain breads, pasta, and rice for health reasons find that over time, their palate adapts, until white breads and rice taste too bland!

October 24

Keeping tight control of your blood sugar level helps prevent and minimize nerve damage. In one trial, patients who received aggressive insulin therapy and maintained reasonably low blood sugar reduced their risk of neuropathy by 60 percent!

1½ tablespoons gingersnap crumbs (2 cookies)

¼ teaspoon ground ginger

2 ounces reduced-fat cream cheese, softened

1 container (6 ounces) peach sugar-free fat-free yogurt

¼ teaspoon vanilla

⅓ cup chopped fresh peach or drained canned peach slices in juice

1. Place cookies and ginger in small resealable food storage bag; crush with rolling pin.

2. Beat cream cheese in small bowl with electric mixer at medium speed until smooth. Add yogurt and vanilla. Beat at low speed until smooth and well blended. Stir in peach.

3. Divide peach mixture between two 6-ounce dessert dishes. Cover and refrigerate 1 hour. Top each serving with half of gingersnap crumb mixture just before serving.

Makes 2 servings

Note: Gingersnaps can also be served whole with the dessert instead of crushed.

Dietary Exchanges: 1 Bread/Starch, 1 Fat, ½ Milk

Calories 148, **Total Fat** 5g, **Saturated Fat** 3g, **Protein** 6g, **Carbohydrates** 18g, **Cholesterol** 16mg, **Dietary Fiber** 1g, **Sodium** 204mg

October 23

If you experience tingling or numbness in your feet, legs, arms, or hands, alert your health care team. Those symptoms may signal diabetic neuropathy, a form of nerve damage. Your risk for developing neuropathy increases if you have a hard time maintaining glucose control, have high blood pressure, smoke, are overweight, or have had diabetes for a long time.

March 25

Are there household tasks that you pay to have done? Consider doing some of them yourself, if time and health permit. Doing chores like cleaning and gardening can burn calories while increasing your insulin sensitivity.

2 large sweet potatoes (about 1¼ pounds), peeled and cut into 1-inch pieces

2 medium parsnips (about ½ pound), peeled and cut into ½-inch slices

¼ cup evaporated skimmed milk

1½ tablespoons butter or margarine

½ teaspoon salt

⅛ teaspoon ground nutmeg

¼ cup chopped fresh chives or green onions

1. Combine sweet potatoes and parsnips in large saucepan. Cover with cold water; bring to a boil over high heat. Reduce heat; simmer, uncovered, 15 minutes or until vegetables are tender.

2. Drain vegetables; return to pan. Add milk, butter, salt and nutmeg. Mash with potato masher over low heat until desired consistency is reached. Stir in chives.

Makes 6 servings

Dietary Exchanges: 1½ Bread/Starch, ½ Fat

Calories 136, **Total Fat** 3g, **Saturated Fat** 2g, **Protein** 3g, **Carbohydrates** 25g, **Cholesterol** 8mg, **Dietary Fiber** 5g, **Sodium** 243mg

March 26

A major clinical study that took place between 1998 and 2001—the Diabetes Prevention Program (DPP)—compared three groups of people who had been diagnosed with prediabetes. One group acted as a control group. Another group took the oral medication metformin. The third group received in-depth training encouraging weight loss through a healthy diet and exercise.

The study found that the group who were taught to make lifestyle changes lowered their risk of developing full-blown diabetes by 58 percent! That was a better result than the group who received metformin, who lowered their risk by 31 percent.

October 21

Seasonal Food Spotlight

Seek out sweet potatoes and you won't be sorry. They have lots of fibers, tons of vitamin A, and good amounts of vitamin C, vitamin B6, and potassium. Research suggests that having a bit of fat with the sweet potato (oil or butter, for example) helps you absorb the full nutritional benefits.

March 27

Like most members of the bean family, fava beans are full of nutritional benefits. Low in fat, they offer large amounts of fiber, protein, iron, and folate. If you don't see them in your grocery, check under the name broad beans instead.

October 20

Lifestyle changes help lower blood pressure, but many people with hypertension need medication. A large study of patients with diabetes in the United Kingdom found that about one-third required three or more medications to keep their blood pressure at a safe level. That sounds daunting, but consider the benefits: The same study found that patients who maintained tight control over their blood pressure reduced their risk of stroke by 44 percent and heart failure by 56 percent. They were also less likely to lose their eyesight, a common complication of hypertension and diabetes.

1 package (about 16 ounces) angel
    food cake mix
½ cup cold water
1 teaspoon almond extract

1 package (14 ounces) sweetened
    flaked coconut, divided
½ cup slivered almonds,
    coarsely chopped

1. Preheat oven to 325°F. Line cookie sheets with parchment paper.

2. Beat cake mix, water and almond extract in large bowl with electric mixer at medium speed until well blended. Add half of coconut; beat until blended. Add remaining coconut and almonds; beat until well blended. Drop dough by tablespoonfuls 2 inches apart onto prepared cookie sheets.

3. Bake 22 to 25 minutes or until golden brown. Cool on cookie sheets 3 minutes. Remove to wire racks; cool completely.

Makes 40 cookies (1 cookie per serving)

Dietary Exchanges: 1 Diabetic Carb Count, 1 Bread/Starch

Calories 94, **Total Fat** 4g, **Saturated Fat** 3g, **Protein** 2g, **Carbohydrates** 14g, **Cholesterol** 0mg, **Dietary Fiber** 1g, **Sodium** 86mg

October 19

Did you know that cholesterol isn't affected just by what you eat? Exercise boosts HDL ("good") cholesterol and produces a small drop in LDL ("bad") cholesterol. Also, a workout reduces the volume of blood your heart pumps and relaxes your blood vessels, leading to lower blood pressure.

March 29

When you eat apples, don't peel them! Paring off the skin of apples or other fruits strips away fiber and nutrients, so leave it on.

8 cups air-popped popcorn (about ⅓ cup kernels)

2 tablespoons honey

4 teaspoons butter

¼ teaspoon ground cinnamon

1. Preheat oven to 350°F. Spray jelly-roll pan with nonstick cooking spray. Place popcorn in large bowl.

2. Combine honey, butter and cinnamon in small saucepan; cook and stir over low heat until butter is melted and mixture is smooth. Immediately pour over popcorn; toss to coat evenly. Pour onto prepared pan.

3. Bake 12 to 14 minutes or until coating is golden brown and appears crackled, stirring twice.

4. Cool popcorn on pan. (As popcorn cools, coating becomes crisp. If not crisp enough, or if popcorn softens upon standing, return to oven and heat 5 to 8 minutes.) Store in airtight container.

Makes 4 servings

Dietary Exchanges: 1 Bread/Starch, 1 Fat

Calories 117, **Total Fat** 4g, **Saturated Fat** 1g, **Protein** 2g, **Carbohydrates** 19g, **Cholesterol** 0mg, **Dietary Fiber** 1g, **Sodium** 45mg

March 30

Cutting down on fat in your diet helps:

- Lower your cholesterol level.
- Keep your heart and blood vessels healthy.
- Control your weight.
- Improve your blood glucose level.

October 17

Women who have not reached menopause have a far lower risk for heart disease than men do, possibly due to the beneficial effects of estrogen. However, having diabetes changes this: Women with diabetes have the same risk for heart disease as men, regardless of their age.

March 31

People who have problems with circulation or nerve damage that affects their lower extremities can still exercise—non-weight-bearing exercises such as stationary cycling, water exercise, or upper-body weight lifting are all options. (As always, talking to your health care providers before beginning an exercise program is a good idea.)

October 16

Drinking plenty of water is important for everyone, but especially for people with diabetes. Your kidneys help lower rising blood sugar levels by excreting excess glucose in urine. But when the body's water supply runs low, your kidneys slow down urine production, and glucose builds up further. Hyperosmolar hyperglycemic syndrome is seen most often with elderly patients with diabetes who may not be able to tend to their own thirst.

2 cans (6 ounces each) tuna packed in water, rinsed and well drained

3 tablespoons light mayonnaise

2 tablespoons fat-free sour cream or fat-free plain yogurt

1 to 1½ tablespoons sugar

1 teaspoon curry powder

¼ teaspoon ground cumin

4 ounces sliced water chestnuts, drained and coarsely chopped

⅛ teaspoon ground red pepper

4 slices cinnamon-raisin bread, lightly toasted and cut in half diagonally

1. Combine tuna, mayonnaise, sour cream, sugar, curry powder and cumin in medium bowl; mix well. Add water chestnuts and red pepper; mix well. Cover and refrigerate 15 minutes to allow flavors to develop.

2. Arrange toast halves on serving plates. Spoon tuna mixture evenly onto toast halves.

Makes 4 servings

Dietary Exchanges: 1½ Bread/Starch, 2 Meat

Calories 233, **Total Fat** 5g, **Saturated Fat** 1g, **Protein** 24g, **Carbohydrates** 22g, **Cholesterol** 31mg, **Dietary Fiber** 2g, **Sodium** 465mg

October 15

Quick Quiz

What is hyperosmolar hyperglycemic syndrome?

A. A dental condition involving the effect
hyperglycemia has on the molars and other teeth

B. A condition that occurs when a person with
diabetes isn't sufficiently hydrated

C. A condition that occurs when a person with
diabetes drinks too much water

D. A condition that occurs when a person with
diabetes drinks too much alcohol

Answer: B. Hyperosmolar hyperglycemic syndrome (HHS) occurs when a person with
diabetes drinks too little water. Early symptoms include weakness, thirst, and fatigue.
Later symptoms include rapid heartbeat, sunken eyeballs, and confusion.

April 2

As the weather warms up, many people turn to outside sports or kick their exercise routine up a notch. Staying active is great, but remember to look after your feet. Invest in good shoes, make sure to wear socks to keep your feet dry, and check your feet daily for injuries.

¾ cup cholesterol-free egg substitute

¼ cup chopped green onions

¼ cup plain fat-free yogurt

2 teaspoons all-purpose flour

1 teaspoon dried basil

⅛ teaspoon salt

⅛ teaspoon black pepper

¾ cup frozen broccoli florets, thawed and drained

1 can (6 ounces) boneless skinless salmon, drained and flaked

2 tablespoons grated Parmesan cheese

1 plum tomato, thinly sliced

¼ cup fresh bread crumbs

1. Preheat oven to 375°F. Spray 1½-quart casserole or 9-inch deep-dish pie plate with nonstick cooking spray.

2. Combine egg substitute, green onions, yogurt, flour, basil, salt and pepper in medium bowl until well blended. Stir in broccoli, salmon and cheese. Spread evenly in prepared casserole. Top with tomato slices and sprinkle with bread crumbs.

3. Bake, uncovered, 20 to 25 minutes or until knife inserted near center comes out clean. Let stand 5 minutes before serving. Cut into wedges before serving.

Makes 4 servings

Dietary Exchanges: 1 Bread/Starch, ½ Fat, 1 Vegetable, 2 Meat

Calories 227, **Total Fat** 6g, **Saturated Fat** 2g, **Protein** 25g, **Carbohydrates** 20g, **Cholesterol** 25mg, **Dietary Fiber** 5g, **Sodium** 717mg

April 3

Protect yourself when you exercise. Test your blood sugar before, during, and after exercise. Carry enough water so that you'll stay hydrated. And wear a bracelet or shoe tag that identifies you as a person with diabetes.

October 13

Stress-buster

If you work at a desk all day, pause every half hour or so to stand, do some stretches, and look away from your computer screen. When you can, take a short, brisk walk during your lunch hour to add some additional activity during your day and remind yourself that there's life outside the office.

April 4

An 11th-century Persian physician, Avicenna, noted that people with diabetes produce "wonderfully sweet" urine. He prescribed the use of herbs, including fenugreek and wormseed.

October 12

Jason Johnson was diagnosed with type 1 diabetes as a child, but he pursued his dream of baseball and made it to the major leagues. In 2004, while playing with the Detroit Tigers, he became the first Major League Baseball player to wear an insulin pump while on the field.

Nonstick cooking spray
1 medium onion, very thinly sliced
1 boneless beef top sirloin steak
   (about 1 pound)

¼ cup water
2 tablespoons Worcestershire sauce
1 tablespoon sugar

1. Lightly coat 12-inch skillet with cooking spray; heat over high heat. Add onion; cook and stir 4 minutes or until browned. Remove from skillet and set aside. Wipe out skillet with paper towel.

2. Coat same skillet with cooking spray; heat over high heat. Add beef; cook 10 to 13 minutes for medium-rare to medium, turning once. Remove from heat and transfer steak to cutting board; let stand 3 minutes before slicing.

3. Meanwhile, return skillet to high heat; add onion, water, Worcestershire sauce and sugar. Cook 30 to 45 seconds or until most liquid has evaporated.

4. Thinly slice beef on the diagonal; serve with onions.

Makes 4 servings

Dietary Exchanges: ½ Bread/Starch, 1 Fat, 3 Meat

Calories 159, **Total Fat** 5g, **Saturated Fat** 2g, **Protein** 21g, **Carbohydrates** 7g, **Cholesterol** 60mg, **Dietary Fiber** 1g, **Sodium** 118mg

2½ cups chopped cooked barbecue chicken*
½ cup corn niblets, roasted**
3 to 4 canned sweet roasted red peppers, chopped
2 green onions, chopped
¼ cup fresh cilantro, minced
2 tablespoons canola oil

2 tablespoons lime juice
1 teaspoon Dijon mustard
⅛ teaspoon black pepper
1 clove garlic, minced
Shredded cabbage (optional)

*Purchase barbecue roasted chicken breasts from the deli and remove the skin.
**Roast whole ear of corn on grill, or place under broiler until browned. Frozen or canned corn niblets can also be used

1. Combine chicken, corn, red peppers, green onions and cilantro in large bowl; gently mix.

2. Combine oil, lime juice, mustard, black pepper and garlic in small bowl; whisk well.

3. Spoon dressing over chicken mixture; carefully blend to bind ingredients.

4. Divide salad mixture into 4 portions; spoon onto shredded cabbage, if desired.

Makes 4 servings (¾ to 1 cup per serving)

Dietary Exchanges: 1 Bread/Starch, 1½ Fat, 1 Meat

Calories 196, **Total Fat** 12g, **Saturated Fat** 2g, **Protein** 11g, **Carbohydrates** 11g, **Cholesterol** 48mg, **Dietary Fiber** 1g, **Sodium** 289mg

April 6

Myth or Fact? Exercise can produce a rise in your blood sugar levels.

Fact. While exercise generally lowers your blood sugar levels and increases insulin sensitivity, it can sometimes work in the opposite way, because intense exercise can cause a surge of the stress hormone adrenaline.

October 10

Acronym Alert: AGE

AGE stands for advanced glycated end products. These are compounds that are produced when glucose and protein interact in your body— everyone develops them, and they accumulate as we age. However, elevated glucose levels means they form at an accelerated rate. High concentrations of these compounds may damage arteries and make them more likely to clog.

April 7

If you experience high blood sugar during exercise, drink plenty of water during and after your workouts. If you experience very high blood sugar—greater than 300 mg/dl, for example—consult your doctor and ask whether you should be checking your urine for ketones. Ketones in the urine mean you are deficient in insulin; do not exercise if your urine contains ketones.

October 9

Don't be afraid to ask your friends for help. Though ultimately you are responsible for managing your diabetes, some friends with extra time and energy may want to help you, and just need a concrete task, whether it's researching pros and cons of different types of meters, meeting for a walk instead of a meal, or just asking you about your progress.

April 8

Cutting Down on Salt

Sandwiches are a staple food for lunches, but bread, cheese, and pre-packaged deli meats can all contain lots of sodium. Check your grocery for low-sodium versions of your sandwich makings, and fill your sandwich and your stomach with vegetables like sliced cucumbers, tomatoes, and lettuce.

October 8

If the leaves are changing colors in your area, gather your family or friends and go on a photo hike. You can even make a game of it, rewarding prizes for photographs of birds you spot, the prettiest tree, and so forth.

2½ cups cocoa-flavored sweetened rice cereal

6 low-fat honey graham crackers, broken into ¼-inch pieces

3 tablespoons margarine

1 tablespoon sucralose-brown sugar blend sweetener

3½ cups mini marshmallows, divided

1 square (1 ounce) semisweet or milk chocolate, melted (optional)

1. Spray 9-inch square baking pan with nonstick cooking spray. Combine cereal and graham cracker pieces in large bowl.

2. Combine margarine and sucralose-brown sugar blend in large microwavable bowl; microwave on HIGH 25 to 30 seconds or until margarine is melted. Add 2½ cups marshmallows; microwave on HIGH 1½ to 2 minutes, stirring after 1 minute, or until marshmallows are melted and smooth.

3. Add marshmallow mixture to cereal mixture; stir to coat. Add remaining 1 cup marshmallows; stir until blended. Press evenly into prepared pan using waxed paper. Cool completely. Drizzle with chocolate, if desired. Cut into squares to serve.

Makes 16 servings

Dietary Exchanges: 1 Diabetic Carb Count, 1 Bread/Starch

Calories 89, **Total Fat** 2g, **Saturated Fat** 1g, **Protein** 1g, **Carbohydrates** 16g, **Cholesterol** 0mg, **Dietary Fiber** 0g, **Sodium** 79mg

2 small Granny Smith apples, peeled, cored and chopped (about 1 cup)
⅓ cup cholesterol-free egg substitute
2 tablespoons imitation bacon bits
½ teaspoon sugar substitute
¼ teaspoon ground cinnamon
4 frozen pancakes
4 teaspoons sugar-free maple syrup

1. Combine apples, egg substitute, bacon bits, sugar substitute and cinnamon in small bowl.
2. Place 2 frozen pancakes on microwavable dish and top each evenly with apple mixture. Microwave on HIGH 3 minutes.
3. Drizzle with maple syrup; top with remaining pancakes. Microwave on HIGH 2 minutes.
4. Serve warm or let cool slightly.

Makes 2 servings

Dietary Exchanges: 2 Bread/Starch, 1 Fat, ½ Fruit

Calories 233, **Total Fat** 4g, **Saturated Fat** 1g, **Protein** 11g, **Carbohydrates** 37g, **Cholesterol** 1mg, **Dietary Fiber** 3g, **Sodium** 655mg

April 10

Shopping tip: When you're buying juice, make sure it's 100 percent juice, with no sugar added. Juice can pack a lot of carbohydrates in just a few ounces, so pay attention to the serving size.

October 6

We've all heard the old saying, "An apple a day keeps the doctor away." Indeed, apples make a heart-healthy snack that contain fiber and antioxidants. Some research has suggested that apples may help regulate blood sugar, too.

April 11

One way to encourage weight loss is to eat smaller portions. Here are some habits that will encourage portion control:

• Don't eat directly from a bag or food container. Measure out what you will eat first.

• Take a little more time when you eat. Sometimes it takes a bit of time for your brain to get the message that your stomach is full.

• Serve your food on a smaller plate or bowl.

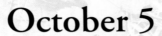

October 5

Cutting Down on Salt

If you keep your salt shaker on the table, move it to the counter. Make adding salt to your meal something you have to think about rather than something you do by habit.

April 12

Quick Quiz

Which seasoning has the most sodium?

A. A tablespoon of soy sauce
B. A tablespoon of olive oil
C. A tablespoon of catsup
D. A tablespoon of margarine

Answer: A. A tablespoon of soy sauce can contain about 1,000 mg of sodium, while olive oil has no sodium, catsup has about 150 mg, and margarine has 140 mg. The American Heart Association recommends no more than 1,500 mg of sodium a day.

October 4

Myth or Fact? Monounsaturated fats actually lower LDL cholesterol.

Fact. The monounsaturated fats found in foods like avocado, most nuts, and olive oil actually lower LDL ("bad") cholesterol.

Raspberry Smoothie

1½ cups fresh or frozen raspberries,
  plus additional for garnish
1 cup plain sugar-free fat-free yogurt
2 packets sugar substitute *or* equivalent of
  4 teaspoons sugar

1 tablespoon honey
1 cup crushed ice
Sprigs fresh mint (optional)

1. Combine 1½ cups raspberries, yogurt, sugar substitute, honey and ice in blender; blend until smooth.

2. Pour into two glasses. Garnish with additional raspberries and mint.

Makes 2 servings

Dietary Exchanges: 1½ Fruit, ½ Milk

Calories 143, **Total Fat** 1g, **Saturated Fat** 1g, **Protein** 8g, **Carbohydrates** 28g, **Cholesterol** 2mg, **Dietary Fiber** 6g, **Sodium** 88mg

¼ cup old-fashioned or quick oats

¼ cup shredded unsweetened coconut

1 package (about 18 ounces) spice cake mix

1¼ cups water

3 eggs *or* 6 egg whites *or* ¾ cup cholesterol-free egg substitute

1 cup solid-pack pumpkin

½ teaspoon ground nutmeg or apple pie spice

½ teaspoon vanilla or vanilla, butter and nut flavoring

1. Preheat oven to 325°F. Line 48 mini (1¾-inch) muffin cups with paper baking cups.

2. Toast oats and coconut in large nonstick skillet over medium heat 3 to 4 minutes or until coconut starts to brown, stirring constantly. Remove from skillet; set aside.

3. Combine cake mix, water and eggs in large bowl. Beat with electric mixer at low speed 30 seconds or until moistened. Beat at medium speed 2 minutes, scraping bottom and side of bowl. Add pumpkin, nutmeg and vanilla; beat until well blended.

4. Spoon batter into prepared muffin cups, filling two-thirds full. Sprinkle oat mixture evenly over top of batter. Bake 10 minutes or until toothpick inserted into centers comes out clean. Cool in pans on wire racks 10 minutes. Remove cupcakes to racks; cool completely. Store in tightly sealed container.

Makes 24 servings

Dietary Exchanges: 1 Bread/Starch, ½ Fat, **Calories** 110, **Total Fat** 3g, **Saturated Fat** 1g, **Protein** 2g, **Carbohydrates** 18g, **Cholesterol** 27mg, **Dietary Fiber** 1g, **Sodium** 175mg

April 14

If you have diabetes, you might have found yourself checking your blood sugar at a strange time or in an unexpected location. IndyCar driver Charlie Kimball and NASCAR driver Ryan Reed, who both have type 1 diabetes, have systems in their racing cars that monitor their blood sugar even while they're going 200 mph!

October 2

Spaghetti squash comes into season in fall and is available through the winter. When cooked, the inside of the squash breaks into long, spaghetti-like strands, which make a yummy, filling substitute for pasta. Low in calories, this member of the squash family provides good fiber, vitamin A, vitamin C, and vitamin B6.

April 15

Stress-buster

Read a funny book, watch a comedy, or engage in an activity that will make you laugh. Laughter is a great stress reliever and helps your body increase circulation and produce painkillers.

October 1

The word insulin comes from the Latin word for "island." That's because insulin, along with some other hormones, is produced by the parts of the pancreas called the islets of Langerhans. Langerhans was a German scientist who discovered those parts of the pancreas in 1869, although he did not understand their function.

April 16

Avocados frequently show up on lists of "superfoods." There's good reason for this— they offer a lot of health benefits! Though they are high in fat, most of that fat is the "good" monounsaturated kind. They also contain healthy amounts of fiber, vitamin C, vitamin K, vitamin B6, folate, and potassium.

September 30

It can be overwhelming to think of anything as a lifelong commitment, including lifestyle changes such as exercising. Focus on manageable, measureable goals—if you can't see yourself committing to exercise each day for the rest of your life, commit to one week. Then renew your commitment each week.

⅔ cup water
⅓ cup uncooked bulgur
1 cup halved grape tomatoes
1 can (6 ounces) tuna packed in water, drained and flaked
¼ cup finely chopped red onion
1 large stalk celery, trimmed and thinly sliced

¼ cup finely chopped avocado
1 tablespoon minced fresh Italian parsley
1 to 2 tablespoons lemon juice
4 teaspoons chicken broth
1 teaspoon olive oil
⅛ teaspoon black pepper

1. Bring water to a boil in small saucepan. Stir in bulgur. Cover; reduce heat to low. Simmer 8 minutes or until bulgur swells and has absorbed most of the water. Remove from heat; cover and let stand 10 minutes.

2. Meanwhile, combine tomatoes, tuna, onion and celery in large bowl. Stir in bulgur, avocado and parsley. Combine lemon juice, broth, oil and pepper in small bowl. Pour over salad. Toss gently to mix. Chill 2 hours before serving.

Makes 3 (1-cup) servings

Dietary Exchanges: 1 Bread/Starch, 1 Meat

Calories 166, **Total Fat** 4g, **Saturated Fat** 1g, **Protein** 17g, **Carbohydrates** 17g, **Cholesterol** 17mg, **Dietary Fiber** 4g, **Sodium** 221mg

September 29

If your body is changing because of diet or exercise, you may have the temptation to hold off on buying new clothes until you reach your "goal weight." But investing in some flattering, well-fitting clothing may give you a positive mental boost that helps you stick to your weight loss plans.

April 18

Diabetes control doesn't happen overnight. It's a process. Accept that you won't be perfect, and don't let feelings of failure discourage you from continuing the process of managing your diabetes.

September 28

When you go to an appointment with a health care provider, write down your concerns, questions, and symptoms, in order of priority, ahead of time. Often, under the pressure of limited time or nervousness during the appointment, you can easily forget questions that seemed clear just the day before.

April 19

If you're having problems with remembering to test your blood glucose levels, do what you can to make the process easy and routine. Consider having two meters, one at home and one at work, to avoid forgetting your meter in one location. Synchronize testing to another activity you perform daily, such as waiting for coffee to brew.

1½ cups orange or vanilla nonfat yogurt

1 can (11 ounces) mandarin orange segments in light syrup, drained and chopped

1 can (8 ounces) pineapple chunks in juice, drained

1 medium banana, sliced

2 tablespoons shredded coconut, toasted

1. Combine yogurt and oranges in medium bowl.

2. Spoon half of yogurt mixture into four serving bowls; top with pineapple. Spoon remaining yogurt mixture over pineapple; top with banana slices. Sprinkle with coconut. Serve immediately.

Makes 4 servings

Dietary Exchanges: 1 Bread/Starch, 2 Fruit

Calories 170, **Total Fat** 1g, **Saturated Fat** 1g, **Protein** 4g, **Carbohydrates** 40g, **Cholesterol** 0mg, **Dietary Fiber** 2g, **Sodium** 60mg

April 20

Go nuts! Nuts contain monounsaturated fats (that's the kind of fat that lowers your "bad" LDL cholesterol). Walnuts are especially healthy, as they contain omega-3 fatty acids that lower heart-disease risk. Do pay attention, though, to portion size and added salt.

September 26

Fear is a common reaction to the stress of dealing with diabetes. While it makes sense to fear the complications of diabetes, you cannot let that fear paralyze you. Instead, let it motivate you to learn all you can about your disease, to monitor your blood sugar tightly, and to gain the best possible control of your glucose levels.

8 ounces small asparagus spears, ends cut off

¼ teaspoon black pepper, divided

1 teaspoon olive oil

5 large egg whites

⅛ teaspoon salt

¹⁄₁₆ teaspoon chipotle chili powder

2 tablespoons minced scallions

¼ cup shredded Parmesan cheese

1 (8-inch) whole wheat tortilla, heated and cut into wedges

1. Preheat oven to 425°F. Place asparagus on baking sheet. Season with ⅛ teaspoon pepper and brush with oil. Roast 15 minutes, or until asparagus are golden brown and tender, shaking baking sheet occasionally. Remove and keep warm.

2. Beat egg whites together until foamy in large bowl. Mix in remaining ⅛ teaspoon pepper, salt, chili powder, scallions and cheese.

3. Coat large skillet with nonstick cooking spray. Pour in egg white mixture. Cook over medium-high heat until edges of omelet are firm and lightly browned. Lift omelet at edges to allow uncooked mixture to pour to the bottom. Continue to cook until egg whites are firm and dry. Cut omelet in half and arrange each half on a plate. Top each with half of asparagus. Divide tortilla wedges between two plates.

Makes 2 servings

Dietary Exchanges: 1 Bread/Starch, 2 Meat, **Calories** 152, **Total Fat** 4g, **Saturated Fat** 1g, **Protein** 15g, **Carbohydrates** 14g, **Cholesterol** 1mg, **Dietary Fiber** 2g, **Sodium** 449mg

September 25

If you've chosen the healthy path to weight loss and have begun including daily exercise along with dietary changes, the bathroom scale may not reflect all the progress you're making, because you may be losing more fat than pounds. Some forms of exercise can add lean mass by building calorie-burning muscles and denser bones. So rather than using the scale alone to gauge your progress, also measure your chest, waist, and hips.

April 22

Do you feel that your health care providers are on your side and knowledgeable about diabetes? If your doctor doesn't have experience treating people with diabetes, or if you dread going to a specific doctor because you feel that he or she acts judgmental or doesn't listen to you, consider switching to another health care provider. Ultimately, you're the boss of your health care team.

½ cup canned fat-free refried beans
4 (8-inch) fat-free flour tortillas
½ cup chunky salsa

4 (¾-ounce) reduced-fat Cheddar cheese sticks

1. Spread beans over tortillas, leaving ½ inch border around edges. Spoon salsa over beans.

2. Place cheese stick on one side of each tortilla. Fold edge of tortilla over cheese stick; roll up. Place burritos, seam side down, in microwavable dish.

3. Microwave on HIGH 1 to 2 minutes or until cheese is melted. Let stand 1 to 2 minutes before serving.

Makes 4 servings

Dietary Exchanges: ½ Bread/Starch, 1 Meat

Calories 109, **Total Fat** 4g, **Saturated Fat** 3g, **Protein** 9g, **Carbohydrates** 11g, **Cholesterol** 10mg, **Dietary Fiber** 4g, **Sodium** 435mg

April 23

One tool that helps people feel in control of their diabetes is visualization. Close your eyes, and see yourself as healthy, active, and in good control of your diabetes.

September 23

Even if you avoid the flu, everyone gets sick sometimes. When you cannot eat or exercise as usual, it can affect your diabetes control. Stress hormones may cause your blood glucose level to go up, while poor appetite or digestive issues may cause your glucose levels to drop. Test your blood glucose levels and your urine for ketones frequently during illness. Talk to your doctor about any over-the-counter medications you take, to discuss potential side effects and to make sure they will not interact with any other medication you are on.

April 24

Most Americans don't eat the recommended amount of fiber, which is unfortunate because it has a long slate of health benefits. Fiber helps control blood sugar, lowers cholesterol, and fills you up without adding calories. It can cause gas, so add fiber into your diet gradually, and stay hydrated.

September 22

Fall is a time of colorful leaves, back-to-school excitement, and the return of football. Unfortunately, it's also the beginning of flu season. The Centers for Disease Control and Prevention recommend that all people with diabetes who are 6 months and older get the flu shot, because diabetes increases the risk of complications that can develop from the flu. (While the flu vaccine is available as both a shot and a nasal spray, CDC guidelines state that people with diabetes should not receive the nasal spray vaccine.) The CDC also recommends the pneumonia vaccine for people with diabetes.

April 25

Some people use fiber supplements to add fiber to their diet. While they can be useful, try to get your fill from fiber-dense foods if you can. Whole-wheat bread, many vegetables, oat bran, legumes, barley, apples, and carrots are all rich in fiber.

September 21

As a general rule of thumb, unripe foods raise blood sugar more slowly than ripe foods. Cold foods raise blood sugar more slowly than hot foods do. And solids raise blood sugar more slowly than liquids do.

April 26

Seasonal Food Spotlight

If you're looking to add fiber to your diet, asparagus is one option! It also contains a long list of vitamins and minerals, including vitamins A, C, K, and E, folate, and manganese.

September 20

Quick Quiz

As a general rule, do raw foods or cooked foods raise your blood sugar more quickly?

    A. Raw foods
    B. Cooked foods

Answer: B. In general, raw foods raise your blood sugar more slowly and cooked foods more quickly.

1 pound fresh asparagus
1 tablespoon olive oil
½ teaspoon salt (optional)
¼ teaspoon black pepper

1 tablespoon balsamic glaze
¼ cup finely shredded or grated
    Parmesan cheese

1. Preheat oven to 375°F.

2. Arrange asparagus in single layer in shallow 11×7-inch baking dish. Drizzle asparagus with oil; gently toss to coat evenly. Sprinkle with salt, if desired, and pepper.

3. Bake 14 to 16 minutes or until crisp-tender. Drizzle balsamic glaze over asparagus; roll again with tongs to coat. Top with cheese.

Makes 6 servings

Dietary Exchanges: 1 Fat, 1 Vegetable

Calories 57, **Total Fat** 3g, **Saturated Fat** 1g, **Protein** 3g, **Carbohydrates** 4g, **Cholesterol** 3mg, **Dietary Fiber** 2g, **Sodium** 53mg

4 cups unsweetened corn cereal squares
2 cups unsalted pretzels
½ cup unsalted pumpkin or squash seeds
1½ teaspoons chili powder
1 teaspoon minced fresh cilantro or parsley

½ teaspoon garlic powder
½ teaspoon onion powder
1 egg white
2 tablespoons olive oil
2 tablespoons lime juice

1. Preheat oven to 300°F. Spray baking sheet with nonstick cooking spray.

2. Combine cereal, pretzels and pumpkin seeds in large bowl. Combine chili powder, cilantro, garlic powder and onion powder in small bowl.

3. Whisk egg white, oil and lime juice in separate small bowl until well blended. Pour over cereal mixture; toss to coat. Add seasoning mixture; mix lightly to coat evenly. Transfer to prepared baking sheet.

4. Bake 45 minutes, stirring every 15 minutes. Cool completely. Store in airtight container.

Makes about 12 servings

Dietary Exchanges: 1 Bread/Starch, ½ Fat

Calories 93, **Total Fat** 3g, **Saturated Fat** 1g, **Protein** 2g, **Carbohydrates** 15g, **Cholesterol** 0mg, **Dietary Fiber** 1g, **Sodium** 114mg

April 28

A lot of us take our cars through a car wash. If you're able, put a little extra movement in your day by washing it yourself!

September 18

Build a little extra activity into your life this week! Sort out a closet of old clothes, suggest a game of Frisbee with some friends, or pledge yourself to going up and down one extra flight of stairs each day.

4 ounces uncooked whole grain penne pasta

4 ounces fresh asparagus spears, trimmed and cut into 2-inch pieces

1½ cups diced cooked chicken breast

½ cup diced red onion

2 tablespoons canola oil

1 tablespoon lemon juice

2 to 3 teaspoons coarse grain Dijon mustard

1 tablespoon chopped fresh tarragon

½ teaspoon salt

¼ teaspoon black pepper

2 ounces reduced-fat blue cheese, crumbled

1. Cook pasta according to package directions, omitting any salt or fat. Stir in asparagus during last 3 minutes of cooking.

2. Meanwhile, combine chicken, onion, oil, tarragon, mustard, salt and pepper in large bowl.

3. Drain pasta and asparagus well. Stir into chicken mixture. Add cheese; stir gently.

Makes 4 servings (about 1½ cups per serving)

Dietary Exchanges: 1 Bread/Starch, ½ Fat, 1 Vegetable, 3 Meat

Calories 293, **Total Fat** 12g, **Saturated Fat** 3g, **Protein** 23g, **Carbohydrates** 24g, **Cholesterol** 48mg, **Dietary Fiber** 4g, **Sodium** 382mg

September 17

When it comes to losing weight, slow, steady, and sustainable works better than any fad or extreme diet. You don't want to lose weight quickly if you're only going to gain it back again as soon as you stop depriving yourself.

April 30

Look back over the month. If there were times that you didn't follow your regimen, can you isolate the factors that led to your slips? Think about your successes, too—what factors helped you achieve success?

September 16

Stress-buster

Think clearly about your commitments. Sometimes we stick with something that's become a hassle out of habit, past the time we get any benefits from it. If someone asks you to take on extra duties at your church, your child's school, or a local organization, don't say "yes" automatically.

May 1

In the United States, May is National Stroke Awareness Month. Diabetes increases the risk of strokes, so make sure that you and your loved ones know the warning signs. The National Stroke Association uses the acronym FAST to help people remember.

Face: Does a person's face droop when he or she smiles?

Arms: Can a person raise both their arms? If one arm drifts downward, that is a warning sign.

Speech: Is a person's speech slurred? Does it make sense?

Time: If a person exhibits stroke symptoms, call 9-1-1 at once.

1½ pounds red potatoes, cut into ½-inch chunks
1 tablespoon plus 1½ teaspoons olive oil, divided
1 red bell pepper, cut into ½-inch pieces
1 yellow or orange bell pepper, cut into
   ½-inch pieces
1 small red onion, cut into ½-inch wedges

2 cloves garlic, minced
½ teaspoon salt
¼ teaspoon black pepper
1 tablespoon balsamic vinegar
¼ cup chopped fresh basil leaves

1. Preheat oven to 425°F. Spray large roasting pan with nonstick cooking spray.

2. Place potatoes in prepared pan. Drizzle with 1 tablespoon oil; toss to coat evenly. Roast 10 minutes.

3. Add bell peppers and onion to pan. Drizzle with remaining oil. Sprinkle with garlic, salt and black pepper; toss to coat evenly. Roast 18 to 20 minutes or until vegetables are browned and tender, stirring once.

4. Transfer vegetables to large serving dish. Drizzle vinegar over vegetables; toss to coat evenly. Add basil; toss again. Serve warm or at room temperature.

Makes 6 servings

Dietary Exchanges: 2 Bread/Starch, ½ Fat

Calories 170, **Total Fat** 4g, **Saturated Fat** 1g, **Protein** 3g, **Carbohydrates** 33g, **Cholesterol** 0mg, **Dietary Fiber** 1g, **Sodium** 185mg

⅔ cup uncooked quinoa

2 cups plus 2 tablespoons fat-free
(skim) milk, divided

⅛ teaspoon salt

¼ cup sugar

1 egg

1½ teaspoons vanilla

2 cups sliced strawberries

¼ cup vanilla yogurt

Ground cinnamon (optional)

1. Place quinoa in fine-mesh strainer; rinse well under cold running water. Combine quinoa, 2 cups milk and salt in medium saucepan. Bring to a simmer over medium heat. Reduce heat to medium-low; simmer, uncovered, 20 to 25 minutes or until quinoa is tender, stirring frequently.

2. Whisk remaining 2 tablespoons milk, sugar, egg and vanilla in medium bowl. Gradually whisk ½ cup hot quinoa mixture into egg mixture, then whisk mixture back into saucepan. Cook over medium heat 3 to 5 minutes or until thickened and bubbly, stirring constantly. Remove from heat. Let cool 30 minutes.

3. Layer quinoa mixture and strawberries in six parfait dishes. Top with dollop of yogurt and sprinkle with cinnamon, if desired.

Makes 6 servings

Dietary Exchanges: 1 Bread/Starch, ½ Fat, ½ Fruit, ½ Milk **Calories** 171, **Total Fat** 2g, **Saturated Fat** 1g, **Protein** 7g, **Carbohydrates** 30g, **Cholesterol** 33mg, **Dietary Fiber** 2g, **Sodium** 105mg

September 14

Diagnosed with type 2 diabetes in his 60s, legendary Blues musician B.B. King didn't let it keep him from continuing to play, tour, and record during the decades that followed.

The list of people with diabetes includes a number of influential and talented musicians, such as Bo Diddley, Ella Fitzgerald, Miles Davis, James Brown, and Dizzy Gillespie.

May 3

In the United States, May is Mental Health Awareness Month. Having a chronic disease like diabetes increases the risk of depression and anxiety. If you're experiencing any of the following symptoms, talk to your doctor and ask for a mental health screening:

A change in sleep patterns

Apathy

Changes in appetite

Loss of energy

Irritation

Feeling, guilty, ashamed, or hopeless

Problems with concentration

Headaches

Upset stomach

September 13

Quick Quiz

What percent of people with type 2 diabetes take insulin?

    A. Insulin is reserved as a treatment
for people with type 1 diabetes
B. 5 percent
C. 40 percent
D. 80 percent

Answer: C. About 40 percent of people with type 2
diabetes take insulin injections.

May 4

The longer name for diabetes is *diabetes mellitus*. The first part of the name comes from the Greek word for "siphon." An English doctor who lived in the 17th century, Thomas Willis, added on the second part of the term, a Latin term meaning "honey sweet."

September 12

Visit your library for audio books you can listen to while you're on the treadmill or exercising. You can slim down while you catch up with your favorite authors.

May 5

Spring is a perfect time to invite your family and friends to share some outdoor activities. Here are a few suggestions:

- Walk through a local farmer's market together.
- Take a hike at a nearby park or forest preserve.
- Go on a family bike ride.

3 tablespoons ketchup
1 tablespoon balsamic vinegar
1 tablespoon olive oil
1½ cups finely chopped onion
1½ cups finely chopped mushrooms
1½ cups chopped baby spinach

1½ pounds extra lean ground sirloin
¾ cup old-fashioned oats
2 egg whites
½ teaspoon salt
½ teaspoon black pepper

1. Preheat oven to 375°F. Spray 6 mini (4¼×2½-inch) loaf pans with nonstick cooking spray. Whisk ketchup and vinegar in bowl until smooth and blended; set aside.

2. Heat oil in large skillet over medium heat. Add onion, mushrooms and spinach; cook and stir 8 minutes or until tender. Remove to large bowl. Let stand until cool enough to handle.

3. Add beef, oats, egg whites, salt and pepper to vegetables; mix well. Divide mixture evenly among prepared pans. Brush half of ketchup mixture evenly over loaves.

4. Bake 15 minutes. Brush with remaining ketchup mixture. Bake 5 minutes or until cooked through (160°F).

Makes 6 servings

Dietary Exchanges: 1 Bread/Starch, 3½ Meat, **Calories** 270, **Total Fat** 11g, **Saturated Fat** 3g, **Protein** 28g, **Carbohydrates** 14g, **Cholesterol** 62mg, **Dietary Fiber** 2g, **Sodium** 362mg

2 cups water
¼ teaspoon salt
1 cup bulgur wheat
1 cup halved cherry tomatoes
1 can (6 ounces) tuna packed in water, drained and flaked
½ cup pitted black niçoise olives

3 tablespoons finely chopped green onions, green part only
1 tablespoon chopped fresh mint leaves (optional)
1½ tablespoons lemon juice, or to taste
1 tablespoon olive oil
⅛ teaspoon black pepper
Mint leaves (optional)

1. Bring water and salt to a boil in medium saucepan. Stir in bulgur. Remove from heat. Cover and set aside 10 to 15 minutes or until water is absorbed and bulgur is tender. Fluff with fork; set aside to cool completely.

2. Combine bulgur, tomatoes, tuna, olives, green onions and chopped mint, if desired, in large bowl. Combine lemon juice, oil and pepper in small bowl. Pour over salad. Toss gently to mix well. Garnish with mint leaves, if desired.

Makes 3 to 4 servings

Calories 307, **Total Fat** 8g, **Saturated Fat** 1g, **Protein** 21g, **Carbohydrates** 40g, **Cholesterol** 17mg, **Dietary Fiber** 10g, **Sodium** 593mg

September 10

Sometimes having an exercise buddy or a healthy-eating buddy can help a lot—it keeps you accountable, and you can give each other tips on what works for you! However, if one person loses weight more quickly than another or if it becomes a competition, the arrangement can turn sour. If an arrangement no longer works for you, don't continue with it just because it worked in the past or you think you should.

May 7

Actress Mary Tyler Moore was diagnosed with type 1 diabetes during the early days of her famous role as Mary Richards in the *The Mary Tyler Moore Show*. She has been very active in raising awareness of the disease, serving as international chairwoman of the Juvenile Diabetes Research Foundation.

September 9

For unpackaged foods that do not have labels, visit the U.S. Government's free nutrient database at:

http://ndb.nal.usda.gov/

You can view nutritional information for thousands of foods.

May 8

Mary Tyler Moore is not the only person with diabetes in show business. Other Hollywood celebrities who deal with the disease include George Lucas, Jean Smart, Tom Hanks, Halle Berry, and Victor Garber.

September 8

Sauces, dressings, and gravies are sources of "cheap" calories—they have high calorie counts without providing many nutrients. Use toppings in moderation, and skip cream-based dressings.

6 hard-cooked eggs, peeled
⅓ cup light mayonnaise
Juice of 1 lemon
1 teaspoon fresh dill, plus
    additional for garnish

¼ teaspoon salt
¼ cup finely chopped green bell pepper
¼ cup finely chopped red bell pepper
2 tablespoons finely chopped red onion
1 English cucumber

1. Slice eggs in half lengthwise; discard yolks. Finely grate or chop egg whites.

2. Whisk mayonnaise, lemon juice, 1 teaspoon dill and salt in medium bowl. Gently stir in egg whites, bell peppers and onion.

3. Cut cucumber in half crosswise; cut each piece in half lengthwise to make 4 equal pieces. Scoop out cucumber pieces with rounded ½ teaspoon, leaving thick shell.

4. Fill each shell evenly with egg white salad. Garnish with additional dill.

Makes 2 servings

Dietary Exchanges: 1½ Fat, 2 Vegetable, 1 Meat

Calories 175, **Total Fat** 9g, **Saturated Fat** 1g, **Protein** 12g, **Carbohydrates** 11g, **Cholesterol** 6mg, **Dietary Fiber** 1g, **Sodium** 756mg

½ package (9 ounces) frozen artichoke hearts

2 cups diced peeled butternut squash

1 cup sliced onion

2 teaspoons extra virgin olive oil

1 package (10 ounces) prepared whole wheat pizza crust

1 cup no-salt-added pasta sauce

¾ cup (3 ounces) shredded part-skim mozzarella and provolone cheese blend

1. Preheat oven to 425°F. Spray baking sheet with nonstick cooking spray. Arrange squash and onion in single layer on prepared baking sheet; drizzle with oil. Bake 25 minutes or until squash is tender. *Increase oven temperature to 450°F.*

2. Meanwhile, prepare artichoke hearts according to package directions. Drain; coarsely chop and set aside.

3. Place pizza crust on pizza pan or baking sheet; spread crust evenly with pasta sauce, leaving 1-inch border. Arrange squash, onion and artichokes on top; sprinkle evenly with cheese.

4. Bake 10 minutes or until cheese is melted. Slice into 6 pieces.

Makes 5 to 6 servings

Dietary Exchanges: 3 Bread/Starch, 1 Fat, 1 Meat

Calories 302, **Total Fat** 9g, **Saturated Fat** 3g, **Protein** 13g, **Carbohydrates** 47g, **Cholesterol** 11mg, **Dietary Fiber** 10g, **Sodium** 444mg

May 10

Myth or Fact? Milk contains sugar.

Fact. While milk doesn't contain sucrose (common table sugar), it does contain a type of sugar called lactose.

September 6

Hypothyroidism (underactive thyroid) is very common among people who have had diabetes for many years. It can make weight loss very difficult. Symptoms include feeling sluggish, decreased appetite, slowed reflexes, constipation, weight gain, and inability to tolerate cold. If you're experiencing those symptoms, talk to your doctor and get screened for a thyroid disorder.

May 11

Cutting Down on Salt

Be sparing with salty condiments such as ketchup, mustard, pickles, and mayonnaise. Try at least one bite of your food plain before adding any condiments, and then just add on a little.

September 5

Cutting Down on Salt

Opt for sweet pickles instead of dill pickles—they generally contain less sodium. Check the nutrition labels on different brands, and select the one containing the least sodium.

May 12

Quick Quiz

Which is more common, type 1 diabetes or type 2 diabetes?

A. Type 1, which accounts for over 9
out of every 10 people with diabetes.
B. Type 1, which accounts for about 7
out of every 10 people with diabetes.
C. They are about equally common.
D. Type 2, which accounts for about 7
out of every 10 people with diabetes.
E. Type 2, which accounts for over 9
out of every 10 people with diabetes.

Answer: E. Type 2 diabetes is much more common than type 1 diabetes.

September 4

Watching any new shows in the new television season? If so, walk while you watch! For a 200-pound person, walking at a slow pace burns about 300 calories per hour. Set up a treadmill in front of the TV, or just walk in place.

4 cups (about 8 ounces) coleslaw mix
½ cup trimmed vertically sliced snow peas
½ cup whole kernel corn (frozen or fresh)
¼ cup low-fat mayonnaise
¼ cup fat-free sour cream

¼ cup nonfat buttermilk
1 tablespoon cider vinegar
2 teaspoons sugar
¼ teaspoon celery seed

1. Combine coleslaw, snow peas and corn in large bowl.

2. Meanwhile, whisk mayonnaise, sour cream, buttermilk, vinegar, sugar and celery seed in medium bowl. Add to coleslaw mixture and mix to combine.

Makes 4 servings (about ¾ cup per serving)

Dietary Exchanges: 3 Vegetable

Calories 85, **Total Fat** 1g, **Saturated Fat** 1g, **Protein** 3g, **Carbohydrates** 17g, **Cholesterol** 3mg, **Dietary Fiber** 2g, **Sodium** 175mg

3 cups fat-free (skim) milk
¾ cup cholesterol-free egg substitute
3 tablespoons sugar substitute*
3 tablespoons unsweetened cocoa powder

2 teaspoons instant decaffeinated
    coffee granules
1½ teaspoons vanilla

*This recipe was tested with sucralose-based sugar substitute

Combine milk, egg substitute, sugar substitute, cocoa, coffee granules and vanilla in blender; blend until smooth. Serve immediately.

Makes 4 servings

Variation: This rich and delicious shake tastes great served over ice, too.

Dietary Exchanges: ½ Bread/Starch, ½ Meat, ½ Milk

Calories 147, **Total Fat** 2g, **Saturated Fat** 1g, **Protein** 13g, **Carbohydrates** 23g, **Cholesterol** 3mg, **Dietary Fiber** 1g, **Sodium** 182mg

May 14

If you're looking for a healthy, versatile veggie, peas are an easy-peasy choice to make! Don't just think of them as a side dish—they also make tasty additions to pasta, casseroles, and salads. Along with antioxidant benefits, peas pack a lot of protein into a small serving, and they're a great source of fiber as well. They contain a lot of vitamins and minerals too, including iron, thiamin, vitamin K, phosphorus, and manganese.

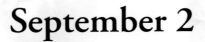

September 2

Myth or Fact? Diabetic retinopathy is the leading cause of blindness in American adults.

Fact. Symptoms of diabetic retinopathy include blurry vision, floaters, night blindness, loss of peripheral vision, and difficulty reading. But because diabetic retinopathy does not always cause symptoms, it's important that people with diabetes have regular eye exams.

May 15

How meat is prepared can be a factor in how much fat you eat. The visible fat you see on meat is saturated fat, so trim it from red meat before cooking. Opt for skinless poultry and trim off visible fat on that as well. And think about the method you're using to cook the meat. Frying, for example, requires added fat—try broiling, roasting, or grilling instead.

September 1

The National Diabetes Information Clearinghouse (http://diabetes.niddk. nih.gov) was created in 1978 by the U.S. federal government, and contains a lot of information and links to resources.

2 tablespoons all-purpose flour
1 teaspoon dried thyme
½ teaspoon salt
¼ teaspoon black pepper
2 teaspoons olive oil
4 large bone-in chicken thighs (1½ to 1¾ pounds), skin removed

1 cup fat-free reduced-sodium chicken broth
12 ounces fresh green beans, trimmed and cut into 1-inch pieces
1 large red bell pepper, cut into short, thin strips
¼ cup grated Parmesan cheese

1. Combine flour, thyme, salt and black pepper in large resealable food storage bag. Add chicken, on piece at a time; shake to coat lightly with flour mixture.

2. Heat oil in large deep skillet over medium heat until hot. Place chicken meat side down in skillet; sprinkle any remaining flour mixture from bag over chicken. Cook 5 minutes; turn chicken over, add broth to skillet. Simmer, uncovered, 15 minutes, turning once.

3. Add green beans and bell pepper to skillet. Cover; simmer 8 to 10 minutes or until vegetables are tender and chicken is cooked through and juices run clear. Transfer chicken to serving plates. Stir vegetable mixture; serve vegetables over chicken. Sprinkle with cheese.

Makes 4 servings

Dietary Exchanges: 2 Vegetable, 2 Meat, **Calories** 178, **Total Fat** 7g, **Saturated Fat** 2g, **Protein** 19g, **Carbohydrates** 11g, **Cholesterol** 68mg, **Dietary Fiber** 3g, **Sodium** 518mg

August 31

A lot of times, food cravings have less to do with being hungry and more to do with other factors. Distract yourself by engaging in a healthy or neutral habit: Chew sugarless gum, do a puzzle online, or make yourself a cup of tea.

May 17

You don't need to cut red meat out of your diet, but take in account how often you eat it and your serving size when you do. Fish contains mostly monounsaturated fat, which is beneficial. Poultry contains more saturated fat than fish, but less than red meat.

August 30

If you have a choice, opt for the white meat when you're eating poultry. It contains less fat than the dark meat. Take the skin off poultry and fowl for an option that's even lower in fat.

May 18

Stress-buster

Diabetes can be isolating, even if your friends and family try to be supportive—and sometimes, unfortunately, they don't know how to be. If you're feeling alone, join a support group for people with diabetes. If a local support group doesn't exist, look for forums online where you can share stories, advice, and understanding.

August 29

Quick Quiz

A gram of fat contains more calories than a gram of carbohydrate

A. True
B. False

Answer: True. Every gram of fat contains nine calories, while a gram of carbohydrate contains just four. So a four-ounce serving of low-fat frozen yogurt might contain 100 calories, while the same amount of full-fat ice cream would contain about 150.

May 19

A strong routine helps diabetes management. As much as possible, stick to your normal schedule for eating and sleeping, even on weekends. If you have a vacation coming up that will make a schedule change necessary, shift your schedule gradually, in the weeks before the vacation.

3 (3-inch) plain rice cakes, broken into
  bite-size pieces
1½ cups bite-size frosted shredded
  wheat cereal
¾ cup pretzel sticks, halved
3 tablespoons reduced-fat margarine, melted

2 teaspoons reduced-sodium
  Worcestershire sauce
¾ teaspoon chili powder
⅛ to ¼ teaspoon ground red pepper

Preheat oven to 300°F. Combine rice cake pieces, cereal and pretzels in 13×9-inch baking pan. Combine margarine, Worcestershire sauce, chili powder and pepper in small bowl. Drizzle over cereal mixture; toss to combine. Bake 20 minutes, stirring after 10 minutes.

Makes 6 (⅔-cup) servings

Dietary Exchanges: 1½ Bread/Starch, ½ Fat

Calories 118, **Total Fat** 3g, **Saturated Fat** 1g, **Protein** 2g, **Carbohydrates** 20g, **Cholesterol** 0mg, **Dietary Fiber** 1g, **Sodium** 156mg

1 eggplant (1¼ pounds), peeled
2 egg whites
½ cup Italian-style panko bread crumbs
Nonstick cooking spray
3 tablespoons reduced-fat chipotle
    mayonnaise

4 whole wheat hamburger buns, warmed
1½ cups loosely packed baby spinach
8 thin slices tomato
4 slices pepper jack cheese

1. Preheat oven to 375°F. Spray baking sheet with cooking spray. Cut 4 slices (½-inch thick) from widest part of eggplant. Beat egg whites in shallow bowl. Place panko on medium plate.

2. Dip eggplant slices in egg whites; dredge in bread crumbs, pressing gently to adhere. Place on prepared baking sheet. Bake 15 minutes or until golden brown; turn and coat with cooking spray. Bake 15 minutes.

3. Spread mayonnaise on bottom halves of buns and top with spinach, tomatoes and eggplant slice. Top with cheese and tops of buns.

Makes 4 servings

Calories 349, **Total Fat** 12g, **Saturated Fat** 3g, **Protein** 16g, **Carbohydrates** 47g, **Cholesterol** 20mg, **Dietary Fiber** 13g, **Sodium** 628mg

August 27

Uncontrolled blood sugar levels make it difficult to control food intake. High blood sugar levels tend to increase appetite, while low blood sugar requires treatment with extra calories. Sometimes medication may be necessary to help people get their blood sugar in a range that allows them to get their eating under control.

May 21

When you go out to dinner with friends, be prepared for a potential change in your schedule. Pack a small snack in case you end up having a difficult time deciding on a restaurant or the food doesn't arrive promptly.

August 26

Sometimes when you change your diet or begin to exercise more, friends or family members may be resistant—they may see the changes you make as an unwelcome judgment of their own habits, or they may expect a change in the friendship. Hold fast to doing what you need to do for the sake of your health. Deep down, people tend to have respect and admiration for those who make the tough choices and care for themselves, as long as they don't force their beliefs on others.

May 22

Myth or Fact? Glucose levels can continue to fall for up to 24 hours after strenuous exercise.

Fact. That's one reason why it's important to test both before and after you exercise.

2 teaspoons vegetable oil
2 teaspoons honey
¼ teaspoon wasabi powder*

1 package (10 ounces) shelled
    edamame, thawed if frozen
Kosher salt (optional)

*This ingredient can be found in the Asian section of most supermarkets and in Asian specialty markets.

1. Preheat oven to 375°F.

2. Combine oil, honey and wasabi powder in large bowl; mix well. Add edamame; toss to coat. Spread on baking sheet in single layer.

3. Bake 12 to 15 minutes or until golden brown, stirring once. Immediately remove from baking sheet to large bowl; sprinkle generously with salt, if desired. Cool completely before serving. Store in airtight container.

Makes 4 to 6 servings

Dietary Exchanges: ½ Bread/Starch, 1 Meat

Calories 78, **Total Fat** 4g, **Saturated Fat** 1g, **Protein** 4g, **Carbohydrates** 7g, **Cholesterol** 0mg, **Dietary Fiber** 1g, **Sodium** 7mg

May 23

Having diabetes doesn't stop a person from being a good driver. But if you're at risk of hypoglycemia, test your blood sugar before driving. Always keep your car stocked with a carbohydrate snack.

August 24

If you're looking for a good source of fiber, reach for a snack of edamame (young soybeans). Edamame is also high in iron, calcium, vitamin K, and potassium. This word is pronounced ed-uh-MAH-may.

2 cups all-purpose flour
1 teaspoon baking powder
1 teaspoon baking soda
½ teaspoon salt
½ cup reduced-fat sour cream
½ cup fat-free (skim) milk

⅓ cup sugar
¼ cup vegetable oil
¼ cup cholesterol-free egg substitute
2 tablespoons lemon juice
1 teaspoon grated lemon peel
3 pints strawberries

1. Preheat oven to 350°F. Coat 8×4-inch loaf pan with nonstick cooking spray; set aside. Combine flour, baking powder, baking soda and salt in large bowl.

2. Combine sour cream, milk, sugar, oil, egg substitute, lemon juice and lemon peel in medium bowl. Stir sour cream mixture into flour mixture until well blended; pour batter into prepared pan.

3. Bake 45 to 50 minutes or until toothpick inserted into center comes out clean. Remove to wire rack to cool completely. Slice cake and serve with strawberries.

Makes 16 servings

Dietary Exchanges: 1 Bread/Starch, 1 Fat, 1 Fruit

Calories 180, **Total Fat** 6g, **Saturated Fat** 1g, **Protein** 4g, **Carbohydrates** 28g, **Cholesterol** 4mg, **Dietary Fiber** 2g, **Sodium** 264mg

August 23

If you'd like to try out a new exercise routine without investing a lot of money in a class or materials, check your local library. They may have DVDs or digital downloads that you can check out to see if something suits you.

May 25

When you test your blood glucose level,
don't just track the numbers—make notes of
your level of activity that day, whether you
ate more or less than normal, or whether
you were sick or not.

August 22

If you're having trouble meeting your goals, write them down. Put them on prominent display on your refrigerator or bathroom mirror.

May 26

Exercising at about the same time each day is best for improving blood sugar control and for sticking with an exercise program over time. But if you need to vary the times of your workouts, don't worry—just be prepared to make adjustments to your insulin or medication as needed.

3 bananas, peeled
6 ice cream sticks or wooden skewers
½ cup semisweet chocolate chips

1½ teaspoons vegetable oil
¼ cup sprinkles, coconut, chopped peanuts or crushed cookies (optional)

1. Line baking sheet with waxed paper or aluminum foil; set aside. Cut each banana in half. Insert ice cream stick halfway into each banana. Place on prepared baking sheet; freeze 1 hour.

2. Stir chocolate chips and oil in small saucepan over low heat until melted and smooth. Place toppings on individual plate, if using; set aside.

3. Remove pops from freezer. Spoon chocolate over each banana while holding over saucepan. Roll in toppings. Return to freezer to harden, about 1 hour. Store in airtight container or plastic freezer bag.

Makes 6 servings

Note: If desired, bananas can be cut into 1-inch pieces, frozen, then dipped in chocolate for individual bites.

Dietary Exchanges: 1 Fat, 1½ Fruit

Calories 132, **Total Fat** 6g, **Saturated Fat** 3g, **Protein** 1g, **Carbohydrates** 23g, **Cholesterol** 0mg, **Dietary Fiber** 2g, **Sodium** 2mg

1 cup reduced-fat biscuit baking mix
¼ cup fat-free (skim) milk
2 tablespoons sugar
1¼ cups fresh raspberries

1 cup diced peeled peaches
2 tablespoons raspberry fruit spread
4 tablespoons thawed frozen
   whipped topping

1. Preheat oven to 425°F. Stir baking mix, milk and sugar in small bowl until smooth and well blended. Drop about 3 tablespoons per biscuit onto ungreased baking sheet. Bake 10 to 12 minutes or until tops are slightly browned. Cool on baking sheet 5 minutes.

2. Meanwhile, combine raspberries and peaches in medium bowl; set aside.

3. Microwave fruit spread in small microwavable bowl on HIGH 15 seconds or until softened.

4. Slice warm biscuits in half. Arrange biscuit bottoms on 4 serving plates. Drizzle ½ teaspoon fruit spread over each biscuit bottom. Top evenly with raspberries and peaches. Replace biscuit tops. Drizzle each shortcake with 1 teaspoon fruit spread; top with 1 tablespoon whipped topping.

Makes 4 servings

Dietary Exchanges: 1 Bread/Starch, 1 Fruit

Calories 205, **Total Fat** 3g, **Saturated Fat** 1g, **Protein** 4g, **Carbohydrates** 42g, **Cholesterol** 0mg, **Dietary Fiber** 4g, **Sodium** 335mg

August 20

Are glucose tablets and gels better for treating hypoglycemia than food sources? Not necessarily—any fast-acting carbohydrate will work. The advantage of glucose tablets and gels, though, is that you won't be tempted to snack on them and deplete your emergency stash.

May 28

SEASONAL FOOD SPOTLIGHT

Fresh apricots make a great snack, and they can be sliced and put on salads, oatmeal, or cereal as well. Apricots are rich in potassium, vitamin A, and fiber.

August 19

Sometimes you might feel as if your body is letting your down. When that happens, give yourself a boost by performing a small, manageable act of self-care. Get a new haircut. Book a massage. Buy a new scarf or a colorful pair of socks.

May 29

You may have heard the term "glycemic index" thrown around, but do you know what it means? The glycemic index measures whether an individual food causes an immediate rise in blood sugar (high glycemic index) or a gradual rise in blood sugar (low glycemic index).

½ cup light mayonnaise
½ cup low-fat buttermilk
2 teaspoons sugar
1 teaspoon celery seed
1 teaspoon fresh lime juice

½ teaspoon chili powder
3 cups shredded coleslaw mix
1 cup shredded carrots
¼ cup finely chopped red onion

Whisk mayonnaise, buttermilk, sugar, celery seed, lime juice and chili powder in large bowl until smooth and well blended. Add coleslaw mix, carrots and onion; toss to coat evenly. Cover and refrigerate at least 2 hours before serving.

Makes 8 servings

Dietary Exchanges: 1 Fat, 1 Vegetable

Calories 59, **Total Fat** 4g, **Saturated Fat** 1g, **Protein** 1g, **Carbohydrates** 6g, **Cholesterol** 3mg, **Dietary Fiber** 1g, **Sodium** 143mg

May 30

Figuring out a food's glycemic index can be tricky, especially if it's prepared and eaten in conjunction with other foods. For example, adding a pat of butter to a potato will cause your blood sugar to rise more gradually than if you'd eaten the potato plain. Pasta that is cooked for a longer time period is absorbed more quickly than pasta cooked *al dente*. So use the glycemic index as a tool if it helps you, but pay more attention to the total amount of carbohydrates you consume.

August 17

On August 17, 1996, swimmer Scott Coleman became the first man with diabetes to swim the English Channel. The swim lasted about ten hours. His support crew traveled in a nearby boat and helped him test his blood during the course of the swim.

2 kiwi fruits
1½ cups strawberries

1 tablespoon orange juice
1 tablespoon pine nuts, toasted

1. Peel kiwis and slice into thin rounds. Arrange on 4 dessert plates.

2. Wash, hull and slice strawberries. Arrange over kiwi slices. Drizzle orange juice evenly over each dish. Top evenly with pine nuts.

Makes 4 (½-cup) servings

Dietary Exchanges: 1 Fruit

Calories 57, **Total Fat** 2g, **Saturated Fat** 0g, **Protein** 1g, **Carbohydrates** 10g, **Cholesterol** 0mg, **Dietary Fiber** 2g, **Sodium** 2mg

August 16

If you inject insulin or other medication and plan to exercise, avoid the muscle areas that you will be using during the activity. For example, if you are playing tennis, avoid your racket arm.

June 1

Until 1889, scientists weren't exactly sure how patients developed diabetes, or which organ or organs were involved. Many suspected the kidneys. Then researchers Oskar Minkowski and Josef von Mering removed a dog's pancreas in an experiment and found that this induced diabetes. They set later scientists on the right track.

August 15

Stress-buster

Being short on sleep is stressful on your body, plus it makes it harder to cope with other kinds of stress. Set yourself up for a good night's sleep. Keep a sleep diary if you're having trouble sleeping, in which you track your evening food and caffeine intake and your nighttime habits. What habits help you sleep well?

June 2

Myth or Fact? A chocolate bar contains fast-acting carbohydrates, making one a good fix for a hypoglycemic episode.

Myth. Unfortunately the fat in chocolate delays the rise of blood sugar levels. When you're suffering from hypoglycemia, opt for simple, fast-acting carbohydrates such as hard candies, milk, sugar cubes, or fruit juice.

1 russet potato (12 ounces), unpeeled
8 ounces yellow summer squash, thinly sliced
8 ounces zucchini, thinly sliced
2 cups frozen bell pepper stir-fry blend, thawed
1 teaspoon dried oregano

½ teaspoon salt
⅛ teaspoon black pepper (optional)
½ cup grated Parmesan cheese or shredded reduced-fat sharp Cheddar cheese
1 tablespoon butter or margarine, cut into 8 pieces

1. Preheat oven to 375°F. Spray 12×8-inch glass baking dish with nonstick cooking spray. Pierce potato several times with fork. Microwave on HIGH 3 minutes. Cut potato into thin slices.

2. Layer half of potato slices, yellow squash, zucchini, bell pepper stir-fry blend, oregano, salt, black pepper, if desired, and cheese in prepared baking dish. Repeat layers. Dot with butter. Cover tightly with foil; bake 25 minutes or until vegetables are just tender. Remove foil; bake 10 minutes more or until lightly browned.

Makes 8 servings

Dietary Exchanges: 1 Bread/Starch, ½ Fat, ½ Meat

Calories 106, **Total Fat** 3g, **Saturated Fat** 2g, **Protein** 4g, **Carbohydrates** 15g, **Cholesterol** 8mg, **Dietary Fiber** 2g, **Sodium** 267mg

1 pound ground chicken
⅓ cup chopped green onions
2 tablespoons Worcestershire sauce
1½ to 2 teaspoons chopped fresh thyme
1 clove garlic, minced

¼ cup Dijon mustard
12 whole wheat dinner rolls, cut in half
2 cups mixed salad greens
1 tomato, cut into 12 thin slices

1. Mix chicken, green onions, Worcestershire sauce, thyme and garlic in large bowl. Shape into 12 (½-inch-thick) patties.

2. Spray large skillet with nonstick cooking spray; heat over medium heat. Cook patties 4 to 5 minutes on each side or until cooked through (165°F).

3. Spread bottom halves of buns with 1 teaspoon Dijon mustard and top with salad greens. Place burgers on greens; top with tomato slices and top halves of buns.

Makes 12 Sliders

Dietary Exchanges: 2 Bread/Starch, 2 Meat

Calories 236, **Total Fat** 9g, **Saturated Fat** 2g, **Protein** 19g, **Carbohydrates** 32g, **Cholesterol** 61mg, **Dietary Fiber** 5g, **Sodium** 555mg

August 13

Quick Quiz

When were the first drugs for diabetes introduced?

    A. Before insulin was
developed, in the 1910s
    B. In the 1940s
    C. In the 1950s
    D. In the 1980s

Answer: C. A class of drug known as *sulfonylureas* was introduced in the 1950s.
This class of drug stimulates the pancreas to make more insulin.

June 4

Cutting Down on Salt

Eat fresh fruit and vegetables when you can, and select frozen vegetables over canned. For comparison, an ear of fresh corn has about 1 mg of sodium, a cup of frozen corn has about 7 mg, and a cup of canned corn has a whopping 350 mg.

August 12

When it comes to food, aim for a mindset of choice, not deprivation. Expand your food palette by seeking out foods you've never tried before. Eat the foods you've always enjoyed in moderation, with an eye to your blood sugar levels. Seek out scrumptious foods that can fit in your meal plan.

June 5

Summer is a time of picnics and potlucks. Plan your food intake for the day accordingly. If you know you're going to be eating food that's high in calories and fat, make your other meals lower in calories and fat. And bring along a heart-healthy dish yourself!

August 11

Because diabetes is a progressive disease, people who originally could manage their diabetes through diet and exercise will likely need to add medication at some point. This can be discouraging, but your goal should not be to avoid medications, but to avoid complications. It's not the number of pills you take, but the glucose levels you achieve.

June 6

Berries in general have antioxidant properties and offer good health benefits, and blueberries have an especially good reputation for lowering your risk of heart disease and cancer. Some studies have shown that blueberries and other berries help with blood sugar regulation.

2 ounces extra-firm tofu
¼ cup finely chopped broccoli
¼ cup thawed frozen shelled edamame
⅓ cup cooked brown rice
1 tablespoon chopped green onion

½ teaspoon low-sodium soy sauce
⅛ teaspoon garlic powder
⅛ teaspoon sesame oil
⅛ teaspoon sriracha or hot chili sauce (optional)

1. Press tofu between paper towels to remove excess water. Cut into ½-inch cubes.

2. Combine tofu, broccoli and edamame in large microwavable mug.

3. Microwave on HIGH 1 minute. Stir in rice, green onion, soy sauce, garlic powder, oil and sriracha, if desired. Microwave 1 minute or until heated through. Stir well before serving.

Makes 1 serving

Dietary Exchanges: 1 Bread/Starch, 1 Fat, 1 Vegetable, 1 Meat

Calories 210, **Total Fat** 7g, **Saturated Fat** 1g, **Protein** 14g, **Carbohydrates** 23g, **Cholesterol** 0mg, **Dietary Fiber** 5g, **Sodium** 118mg

2 cups water
1 cup quick-cooking oats
4 tablespoons pourable sugar substitute*
½ teaspoon ground cinnamon
⅛ teaspoon salt
¾ cup fat-free half-and-half

3 tablespoons pourable sugar substitute*
½ teaspoon vanilla extract
½ teaspoon almond extract
1½ cups fresh or frozen blueberries, thawed
½ cup fresh or frozen raspberries, thawed

*This recipe was tested using sucralose-based sugar substitute.

1. Bring water to a boil in large saucepan over high heat. Stir in oats, then reduce heat to medium and cook, uncovered, 2 minutes or until thickened. Remove from heat, stir in 1 tablespoon sugar substitute, cinnamon and salt.

2. Meanwhile, combine half-and-half, 3 tablespoons sugar substitute, vanilla extract, and almond extract in medium bowl to make Sweet Cream.

3. To serve, pour Sweet Cream over oatmeal and top with berries.

Makes 4 servings (½ cup oats, ¼ cup Sweet Cream and ½ cup berries per serving)

Dietary Exchanges: 1 Bread/Starch, ½ Fat, 1 Fruit

Calories 150, **Total Fat** 2g, **Saturated Fat** 1g, **Protein** 5g, **Carbohydrates** 30g, **Cholesterol** 8mg, **Dietary Fiber** 5g, **Sodium** 120mg

August 9

One obstacle that can get in the way of doing what you need to do to manage your diabetes is your self-image—you may have never thought of yourself as an "active person" or a "healthy eater." Start applying these terms to yourself, and see good things start to happen!

June 8

Sometimes people confuse feelings of thirst for hunger. Before reaching for food, enjoy a large glass of water, hot tea, or another calorie-free or low-calorie beverage before reaching for a snack. You may find you were really just thirsty.

August 8

Figs are very good for you. They have plenty of potassium, which is good for blood pressure regulation. They're also full of fiber.

June 9

If you don't have one, consider purchasing a pedometer. A basic pedometer can be found for about $20. Keep track of how many steps you take on a normal day, and then make it a game to see how many extra steps you can fit into your day. Apps that track walking are available as well.

August 7

Cutting Down on Salt

Be aware that "light" salad dressings often have more sodium—and sugar!—than full-fat dressings. Rather than pouring dressing directly on salads, put it on the side. Dip your fork tines into the dressing, then take a bite of salad.

June 10

Sometimes when you're working to lose weight, you'll hit a plateau where you can't seem to lose any more pounds. When this happens, sometimes the solution is to take in more rather than fewer calories. If you take in too few calories, your body may think it is starving and slow down your metabolic rate. Try taking in a few more calories each day to see if your metabolic rate resets.

2 teaspoons olive oil
Nonstick cooking spray
1 large onion, thinly sliced
¼ teaspoon garlic salt
1 package (20 ounces) lean ground turkey

1½ tablespoons Dijon mustard
¼ cup reduced-fat crumbled blue cheese
4 lettuce leaves, torn into 12 pieces
6 whole wheat mini sandwich thin rounds, split and toasted

1. Heat oil in large nonstick skillet over medium-high heat. Add onion; cook and stir 3 minutes. Reduce heat to medium; cook onion 10 minutes or until golden brown, stirring frequently.

2. Mix garlic salt into ground turkey. Shape turkey into 12 (¼-inch-thick) patties.

3. Spray large skillet with nonstick cooking; heat over medium heat. Cook burgers in batches 3 minutes on each side or until cooked through.

4. Combine mustard and blue cheese in small bowl. Place 1 lettuce leaf on bottom of each sandwich thin; top with burger, blue cheese mixture and onions.

Makes 6 servings (12 burgers)

Dietary Exchanges: 1½ Bread/Starch, 3 Meat

Calories 276, **Total Fat** 11g, **Saturated Fat** 3g, **Protein** 24g, **Carbohydrates** 23g, **Cholesterol** 72mg, **Dietary Fiber** 6g, **Sodium** 423mg

June 11

Many people with diabetes can drink alcohol, but be cautious: To your body, alcohol is a toxin. Before you drink, consider alcohol's interaction with any medication you're on. Don't drink on an empty stomach. Drink slowly. And limit yourself to one or two drinks.

August 5

One way to take care of your feet is to lower the temperature of your water tank to 120 degrees Fahrenheit. Your bath water should be about 90 degrees. Test water temperature with your elbow before putting your feet in the bathtub. Your feet may not be as sensitive, and you could burn them.

June 12

Quick Quiz

Alcohol has this effect on the liver:

    A. It forces the liver to release more blood glucose.
    B. It blocks the liver from releasing blood glucose.

Answer: B. While the liver is processing alcohol, it does not release blood glucose if your level drops. So drinking can put you at risk for a hypoglycemic reaction.

August 4

When you're buying shoes, always make sure they're comfortable from the start, to avoid developing blisters while you "break in" a pair of shoes. Feet tend to swell during the day, so go shopping in the afternoon or evening to get a comfortable fit.

4 lean white fish fillets (about 1 pound), such as orange roughy or sole

2 tablespoons plus 2 teaspoons lemon juice, divided

½ teaspoon paprika

1 cup finely chopped seeded tomatoes

2 tablespoons capers, rinsed and drained

2 tablespoons finely chopped fresh parsley

1½ teaspoons dried basil

2 teaspoons olive oil

¼ teaspoon salt

1. Preheat oven to 350°F. Coat 12×8-inch glass baking pan with nonstick cooking spray. Arrange fish fillets in pan; drizzle 2 tablespoons lemon juice over fillets and sprinkle with paprika. Cover with foil; bake 18 minutes or until opaque in center and flakes easily when tested with fork.

2. Meanwhile, in medium saucepan, combine tomatoes, capers, parsley, remaining 2 teaspoons lemon juice, basil, oil and salt. Five minutes before fish is done, place saucepan over high heat. Bring to a boil. Reduce heat and simmer 2 minutes or until hot. Remove from heat.

3. Serve fish topped with tomato mixture.

Makes 4 servings

Dietary Exchanges: 1 Vegetable, 3 Meat

Calories 150, **Total Fat** 4g, **Saturated Fat** 1g, **Protein** 24g, **Carbohydrates** 4g, **Cholesterol** 42mg, **Dietary Fiber** 1g, **Sodium** 360mg

August 3

Myth or Fact? Having diabetes doubles your risk for foot disease.

Fact. People with diabetes are more likely to develop foot problems due to damaged nerves and/or poor circulation caused by high blood sugar. Always take any injuries to your feet seriously.

June 14

Stress-buster

Sometimes our brains get stuck in a cycle of negative thoughts when we try to think through a problem, and instead of solving it we just get more distressed. When your thoughts start going in fruitless circles, give yourself a break. Engage in an activity that will focus your thoughts in other direction. Exercise is one great way to divert your brain—it improves blood flow to the brain, so it may help you come up with a solution when you least expect it!

2½ tablespoons sliced almonds
2½ tablespoons chopped walnuts
3 cups vanilla nonfat Greek yogurt
1⅓ cups sliced strawberries
 (about 12 medium)

2 bananas, cut in half and
 sliced lengthwise
½ cup drained pineapple tidbits

1. Spread almonds and walnuts in single layer in small heavy skillet. Cook and stir over medium heat 2 minutes or until lightly browned. Immediately remove from skillet; cool completely.

2. Spoon yogurt into four bowls. Top with strawberries, banana slices and pineapple. Sprinkle with toasted nuts.

Makes 4 servings

Dietary Exchanges: 1 Fat

Calories 268, **Total Fat** 5g, **Saturated Fat** 1g, **Protein** 10g, **Carbohydrates** 50g, **Cholesterol** 0mg, **Dietary Fiber** 5g, **Sodium** 112mg

½ cup uncooked quinoa
1 cup water
½ teaspoon salt, divided
1 tablespoon olive oil
1 red bell pepper, chopped
⅓ cup chopped green onions

⅛ teaspoon black pepper
⅛ teaspoon dried thyme
1 tablespoon butter
8 plum tomatoes, halved lengthwise, seeded, hollowed out

1. Preheat oven to 325°F. Place quinoa in fine-mesh strainer; rinse well under cold running water. Bring 1 cup water and ¼ teaspoon salt to a boil in small saucepan; stir in quinoa. Cover and reduce heat to low; simmer 12 to 14 minutes or until quinoa is tender and water is absorbed.

2. Heat oil in large skillet over medium-high heat. Add bell pepper; cook and stir 7 to 10 minutes or until tender. Stir in quinoa, green onions, remaining ¼ teaspoon salt, black pepper and thyme. Add butter; stir until melted. Remove from heat.

3. Arrange tomato halves in 13×9-inch baking dish. Fill with quinoa mixture. Bake 15 to 20 minutes or until tomatoes are tender.

Makes 8 servings

Dietary Exchanges: 1½ Bread/Starch, ½ Fat, 1 Vegetable, **Calories** 95, **Total Fat** 4g, **Saturated Fat** 1g, **Protein** 6g, **Carbohydrates** 13g, **Cholesterol** 4mg, **Dietary Fiber** 3g, **Sodium** 165mg

August 1

Dr. Elliot Joslin (1889-1962) was an influential doctor who specialized in diabetes and founded the Joslin Diabetes Center that still exists today. He urged patients to control their glucose levels through diet and exercise. In the early days of insulin treatment, nurses from his institution were instrumental in going out into the surrounding areas to teach patients the basics of self-care and insulin injection.

June 16

In June 2014, news sources reported on a "bionic pancreas" that was being developed and tested. The system, devised for people with type 1 diabetes, tracks blood sugar through a smartphone app and releases insulin or glucagon accordingly.

July 31

High blood sugar doesn't just affect your blood. Extra sugar in the bloodstream leads to *glycosylation* of connective tissues, in which sugar coats tendons and ligaments, limiting their ability to stretch properly. Muscle stiffness, strains, and pulls can result.

June 17

Diabetes didn't keep these athletes from the Olympic podium!

Gary Hall, Jr.—This American swimmer won ten medals (five gold, three silver, two bronze) in the 1996, 2000, and 2004 Olympic Games.

Keith Hansen—Hansen was a member of the 2008 U.S. men's volleyball team that brought home gold from Beijing.

Sir Stephen Redgrave—This British rower won six Olympic medals, five of them gold, over the course of five different Olympic Games.

2 cups water
2 packages (4-serving size each) sugar-free lemon-flavored gelatin
1 teaspoon vegetable oil

1½ cups thawed frozen fat-free whipped topping
1 very firm Granny smith apple, peeled and diced
Fresh mint leaves (optional)

1. Bring water to a boil in large saucepan. Add gelatin; stir until gelatin is completely dissolved. Cover and refrigerate 1 hour.

2. Meanwhile, brush 1-quart gelatin mold or glass bowl with oil.

3. Stir whipped topping into gelatin. Fold in apple. Spread into prepared mold. Cover and refrigerate 4 hours.

4. To unmold, run small metal spatula or pointed knife around edge of mold. Dip bottom of mold briefly into warm water. Place serving plate on top of mold. Invert mold and plate and shake to loosen gelatin. Gently remove mold. To serve, slice into 6 wedges. Garnish with mint.

Makes 6 servings

Dietary Exchanges: ½ Fruit

Calories 64, **Total Fat** 1g, **Saturated Fat** 0g, **Protein** 1g, **Carbohydrates** 11g, **Cholesterol** 0mg, **Dietary Fiber** 1g, **Sodium** 89mg

June 18

Most people underestimate their food intake by 20 percent or more. Food diaries can help you become more aware of what you're actually eating.

July 29

Insulin resistance can set in quickly—even in people who are usually very active, a couple of days without much activity will result in some degree of insulin resistance.

1 large ripe firm banana
½ teaspoon melted butter
2 tablespoons fat-free reduced-sugar
    chocolate syrup

½ teaspoon orange liqueur (optional)
⅔ cup sugar-free vanilla ice cream
2 tablespoons sliced almonds, toasted

1. Spray grid with nonstick cooking spray. Prepare grill for direct cooking.

2. Cut unpeeled bananas lengthwise; brush melted butter over cut sides. Grill bananas, cut side down, over medium-hot coals 2 minutes or until lightly browned; turn. Grill 2 minutes or until tender.

3. Combine syrup and liqueur, if desired, in small bowl.

4. Cut bananas in half crosswise; carefully remove peel. Place 2 pieces banana in each bowl; top with ⅓ cup ice cream, 1 tablespoon chocolate syrup and 1 tablespoon almonds; serve immediately.

Makes 2 servings

Dietary Exchanges: 1 Bread/Starch, 1 Fat, 1½ Fruit,

Calories 198, **Total Fat** 5g, **Saturated Fat** 1g, **Protein** 5g, **Carbohydrates** 33g, **Cholesterol** 3mg, **Dietary Fiber** 2g, **Sodium** 59mg

July 28

Kidney failure is one of the most common complications of diabetes. High glucose levels over time affect your kidneys' ability to filter out waste. To help keep your kidneys healthy:

- Don't smoke.

- Avoid medications that can cause damage to your kidneys.

- Keep your blood glucose controlled.

- Maintain a normal blood pressure.

June 20

Acronym Alert: PIR

PIR stands for psychological insulin resistance. Many people with diabetes resist the idea of taking insulin, even when it's recommended by their doctors. If your doctor has brought up the idea of insulin and you've put it off, don't dismiss it out of hand. Instead, discuss your concerns with your doctor and diabetes educator. Taking insulin may be less daunting than you fear!

Cherry Tomato Pops

4 part-skim mozzarella string cheese sticks
    (1 ounce each)
8 cherry tomatoes
3 tablespoons fat-free ranch dressing

1. Slice cheese sticks in half lengthwise. Trim stem end of each cherry tomato and remove pulp and seeds.

2. Press end of cheese stick into hollowed tomato to make cherry tomato pop. Serve with ranch dressing for dipping.

Makes 8 pops

Dietary Exchanges: ½ Vegetable, ½ Meat

Calories 56, **Total Fat** 3g, **Saturated Fat** 2g, **Protein** 3g, **Carbohydrates** 4g, **Cholesterol** 10mg, **Dietary Fiber** 1g, **Sodium** 210mg

June 21

Did you know that there's a term for the fear of needles and sharp objects? That fear is called belonephobia. People who take insulin who suffer from belonephobia may want to look into insulin "pens," jet injectors, or inhalers.

July 26

You don't need to join a gym or buy a set of weights to get started with strength training! You can use cans, bottles, rolls of coins, or anything else that is small, dense, and easy to grip. Gradually increase the weight and the number of repetitions you do.

June 22

If your family or friends suspect you are having a hypoglycemic episode, have them ask you a question that requires you to think or problem-solve. That will help you and them make an accurate judgment of your condition.

July 25

Fat cells are metabolically stagnant—they don't burn calories when your body is at rest. Muscle cells do. Converting fat to muscle through strength-training (weight lifting) exercises means you'll be burning up more calories even when you aren't actively exercising. Do talk to a doctor before beginning a strength-training program, especially if you have diabetic retinopathy or another condition that might be worsened by straining. And meet with an exercise physiologist or fitness specialist to learn proper technique!

½ (4-serving-size) package vanilla
   sugar-free instant pudding and
   pie filling mix
1¼ cups fat-free (skim) milk
½ cup cubed mango

2 large strawberries, sliced
3 sugar-free shortbread cookies, crumbled
   or 2 tablespoons reduced-fat granola
Strawberry slices (optional)

1. Prepare pudding according to package directions using 1¼ cups milk.

2. Layer one quarter of pudding, half of mango, half of strawberries and one quarter of pudding in parfait glass or small glass bowl. Repeat layers in second parfait glass. Refrigerate 30 minutes.

3. Just before serving, top with cookie crumbs and garnish with strawberries.

Makes 2 servings

Dietary Exchanges: 2 Bread/Starch, ½ Milk

Calories 153, **Total Fat** 1g, **Saturated Fat** 1g, **Protein** 6g, **Carbohydrates** 29g, **Cholesterol** 3mg, **Dietary Fiber** 2g, **Sodium** 129mg

July 24

Sometimes maintaining good habits can seem monotonous. So don't forget to give yourself rewards! Take yourself out to a movie, set aside time to read a good book, invest in shiny gold star stickers for your logbook—do whatever encourages you to keep going over time.

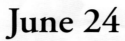

June 24

If you're going to a summer picnic or party, decide ahead of time how you will handle any special foods. For example, will you eat dessert and take extra insulin to compensate?

½ cup (4 ounces) light cream cheese, softened
1 tablespoon honey
¼ teaspoon ground red pepper

2 cups thawed frozen fat-free whipped topping
6 peaches, halved and pits removed
¼ cup slivered almonds, toasted

1. Prepare grill for direct cooking over medium-high heat. Spray grid with nonstick cooking spray.

2. Gently stir cream cheese in medium bowl until smooth. Whisk in honey and ground red pepper until well blended. Fold in whipped topping. Cover and refrigerate until ready to use.

3. Place peaches, cut sides down, on prepared grill. Grill, covered, 2 to 3 minutes. Turn over; grill 2 to 3 minutes or until peaches begin to soften. Remove to plate; let stand to cool slightly.

4. Arrange 2 peach halves, cut sides up, on 6 serving plates. Top evenly with spicy cream cheese topping and almonds. Garnish with mint.

Makes 6 servings

Dietary Exchanges: 1 Bread/Starch, 1 Fat, 1 Fruit

Calories 182, **Total Fat** 6g, **Saturated Fat** 2g, **Protein** 4g, **Carbohydrates** 28g, **Cholesterol** 13mg, **Dietary Fiber** 3g, **Sodium** 107mg

June 25

When you travel and you're determining how much medication, insulin, testing supplies, etc., to bring, a good rule of thumb is to pack twice as many supplies as you think you will use. Pack supplies and snacks such as crackers and raisins in your carry-on items, not your checked luggage.

July 22

Volunteering can be a great way to add some positive energy to your life. Some people find it empowering to volunteer for organizations that raise awareness and money for diabetes and diabetes research. Others may want to take a break from thinking of diabetes by volunteering for another cause they support.

June 26

If you keep a printed logbook to keep track of your blood glucose level and food intake, color-coding is an easy way to help you spot patterns. Highlight low numbers in one color and high numbers in another. Then see what patterns you spot.

July 21

When you're feeling overwhelmed, break down a big task on your to-do list into several smaller ones that are more manageable. Let's say you have to find a new doctor because yours is retiring. Break that down into asking friends or colleagues for recommendations, checking which doctors are in your insurance network, and verifying that your choice has experience with people with diabetes. You'll build momentum with each item that is ticked off the list.

3 cups low-fat plain yogurt, drained*
1 can (4 ounces) green chilies, drained and chopped
¼ cup salsa
¼ cup finely chopped cilantro
¼ cup finely chopped green onions
1 tablespoon lime juice
1 teaspoon dried oregano

1 teaspoon ground cumin
⅛ teaspoon salt
⅛ teaspoon pepper
6 cups assorted cut-up vegetables, such as baby carrots, cauliflower or broccoli florets, celery sticks, grape tomatoes, cucumbers, zucchini sticks

*Place yogurt in a coffee filter or cheesecloth-lined sieve over a bowl and let stand for 3 hours to drain

1. Combine yogurt, chiles, salsa, cilantro, green onions, lime juice, oregano and cumin in medium bowl. Cover and refrigerate 15 minutes. Stir in salt and pepper, if desired.

2. Serve dip with vegetables.

Makes 6 servings

Dietary Exchanges: ½ Fat, 2 Vegetable, ½ Milk

Calories 111, **Total Fat** 2g, **Saturated Fat** 1g, **Protein** 8g, **Carbohydrates** 16g, **Cholesterol** 7mg, **Dietary Fiber** 3g, **Sodium** 281mg

July 20

Seasonal Food Spotlight

Here's an earful about corn! It's loaded with fiber, iron, and vitamin B6. Try seasoning corn on the cob with herbs instead of salt, and olive oil instead of butter.

June 28

If you spot a pattern of high blood glucose levels at bedtime, look at what you ate for dinner. Do certain foods cause your blood glucose level to go up? Can you balance that expected effect by eating less of those foods, exercising before or after that meal, or taking extra insulin or medication?

2 tablespoons reduced-fat mayonnaise
½ teaspoon chili powder
½ teaspoon grated lime peel

4 ears corn, shucked
2 tablespoons grated Parmesan cheese

1. Prepare grill for direct cooking. Combine mayonnaise, chili powder and lime peel in small bowl; set aside.

2. Grill corn over medium-high heat, uncovered, 4 to 6 minutes or until lightly charred, turning 3 times. Immediately spread mayonnaise mixture over corn. Sprinkle with cheese.

Makes 4 servings

Dietary Exchanges: 1 Bread/Starch, ½ Fat

Calories 96, **Total Fat** 4g, **Saturated Fat** 1g, **Protein** 3g, **Carbohydrates** 15g, **Cholesterol** 5mg, **Dietary Fiber** 2g, **Sodium** 104mg

June 29

It's tempting to go barefoot in summer, or to wear flimsy sandals, but remember to protect your feet from bumps, nicks, and bruises that can create big problems later on.

July 18

H.G. Wells, the famous science fiction author who wrote the classics *The War of the Worlds, The Time Machine,* and *The Invisible Man,* had diabetes. He was one of the founders of The Diabetic Association, a British charity organization that exists today as Diabetes UK. (www.diabetes.org.uk)

Other well-known authors with diabetes include Ernest Hemingway and Laura Ingalls Wilder.

1 ripe pineapple, cut into cubes
(about 4 cups)
⅓ cup frozen limeade concentrate

1 to 2 tablespoons fresh lime juice
1 teaspoon grated lime peel

1. Arrange pineapple in single layer on large baking sheet; freeze at least 1 hour or until very firm.*

2. Combine frozen pineapple, limeade concentrate, lime juice and lime peel in food processor or blender; process until smooth and fluffy. If mixture doesn't become smooth and fluffy, let stand 30 minutes to soften slightly; repeat processing. Serve immediately.

Pineapple can be frozen up to 1 month in resealable freezer food storage bags.

Makes 8 servings

Note: This dessert is best if served immediately, but it can be made ahead, stored in the freezer and then softened several minutes before being served.

Dietary Exchanges: 1 Fruit

Calories 56, **Total Fat** 1g, **Saturated Fat** 1g, **Protein** 1g, **Carbohydrates** 15g, **Cholesterol** 0mg, **Dietary Fiber** 1g, **Sodium** 1mg

July 17

Don't just use your grill for hamburgers, steaks, and hot dogs. Portabella mushrooms, corn on the cob, green beans, and other veggies taste great on the grill!

July 1

Don't fall short on supplies! Inventory necessary supplies, such as testing strips or glucose tablets, regularly, and don't let them get too low. You might want to make it something you do on the first day of each month.

July 16

Add pieces of fruit to a cold pitcher of water for an easy, healthy, and refreshing summer drink.

July 2

We've come a long way! In the early 1900s, before insulin was discovered, doctors tried to help their patients with diabetes by restricting carbohydrates. One well-known physician, Frederick Allen, proposed what was basically a starvation diet. A 1915 book that relied on his methodology, called *The Starvation Treatment of Diabetes*, describes the use of "thrice-boiled vegetables" and suggests recipes and meal plans. A sample meal plan for one day was egg, asparagus, and lettuce for breakfast; egg, cauliflower, and lettuce for dinner; and egg, string beans, and celery for supper.

1½ cups fresh raspberries
1 cup fresh blackberries
1 cup fresh blueberries
1 tablespoon fresh lemon juice
3 tablespoons frozen pineapple juice
    concentrate, divided

5 tablespoons all-purpose flour, divided
¾ cup old-fashioned oats
¼ cup walnuts, finely chopped
3 tablespoons packed brown sugar
½ teaspoon ground cinnamon
2 tablespoons melted butter or margarine

1. Preheat oven to 375°F. Spray 8-inch square glass or ceramic baking dish with nonstick cooking spray.

2. Combine berries, lemon juice and 2 tablespoons pineapple juice in medium bowl. Sprinkle with 2 tablespoons flour; toss gently. Spoon into baking dish; set aside.

3. Combine oats, walnuts, brown sugar, cinnamon, remaining 3 tablespoons flour and 1 tablespoon pineapple juice in small bowl. Pour butter over oat mixture; mix until moistened. Spoon over fruit mixture.

4. Bake about 30 minutes or until topping is golden brown and fruit is hot. Serve warm.

Makes 6 servings

Dietary Exchanges: 1 Bread/Starch, 2 Fat, 1 Fruit

Calories 212, **Total Fat** 9g, **Saturated Fat** 2g, **Protein** 4g, **Carbohydrates** 33g, **Cholesterol** 11mg, **Dietary Fiber** 5g, **Sodium** 33mg

July 3

The same 1915 book describes patients initiating the diet under the guidance of the hospital. Before beginning the diet, patients would fast until their urine was free of sugar. During that time, no food was allowed, but the patient was able to drink water and carefully measured quantities of whiskey and black coffee. The book notes, however, that "the whiskey is not an essential part of the treatment."

July 14

If you're taking a road trip, remember to pack carbohydrate-boosting snacks in case you're in need of a fast-acting sugar. If you take insulin, don't leave it in the car unprotected while you sightsee. Use an insulated travel pack to store it safely. Even if insulin doesn't look any different, it may lose some of its effectiveness if exposed to temperature changes.

Breakfast Pom Smoothie

1 small ripe banana
½ cup mixed berries

¾ cup pomegranate juice
⅓ to ½ cup soymilk or milk

Combine banana and berries in blender; process until smooth. Add juice and soymilk; process until smooth. Serve immediately.

Makes 1 (1½ cup) serving

Variations: You can substitute pomegranate-blueberry juice or any other pomegranate juice blend for the pomegranate juice. You can also substitute yogurt for the soymilk.

Dietary Exchanges: 1 Bread/Starch, 3 Fruit

Calories 253, **Total Fat** 1g, **Saturated Fat** 1g, **Protein** 3g, **Carbohydrates** 59g, **Cholesterol** 0mg, **Dietary Fiber** 6g, **Sodium** 35mg

July 13

Stress-buster

Progressive muscle relaxation is a great, quick technique that encourages your muscles to relax. Just tighten and release your muscles one group at a time, from your face to your feet. Spend about ten seconds on each group of muscles.

July 5

Cutting Down on Salt

At restaurants, ask that your food
be prepared without added salt or
monosodium glutamate (MSG).

July 12

Quick Quiz

Which of the following foods contain cholesterol?

      A. Oranges
      B. Kidney beans
      C. Egg salad
      D. Potatoes
      E. All of the above

Answer: C. As an animal product, eggs contain cholesterol.
Only animal products contain cholesterol.

July 6

If you're trying to lose weight, don't give in to the temptation to skip meals. Having regular, evenly-spaced meals will help your body regulate its appetite. Skipping meals tends to cause cravings and hunger that work against your goals.

4 boneless skinless chicken breasts
(about 4 ounces each)

½ cup pitted prunes

½ cup assorted pitted olives (black, green
and/or a combination)

¼ cup light white grape juice or white wine

2 tablespoons olive oil

1 tablespoon capers

1 tablespoon red wine vinegar

1 teaspoon dried oregano

1 clove garlic, minced

½ teaspoon chopped fresh parsley,
plus additional for garnish

2 teaspoons packed brown sugar

1. Preheat oven to 350°F.

2. Place chicken in 8-inch baking dish. Combine prunes, olives, grape juice, oil, capers, vinegar, oregano, garlic and ½ teaspoon parsley in medium bowl. Pour evenly over chicken. Sprinkle with brown sugar.

3. Bake 25 to 30 minutes or until no longer pink in center, basting with sauce halfway through. Garnish with additional parsley.

Makes 4 servings

Dietary Exchanges: 1 Fat, 1 Fruit, 3 Meat

Calories 280, **Total Fat** 11g, **Saturated Fat** 2g, **Protein** 25g, **Carbohydrates** 20g, **Cholesterol** 72mg, **Dietary Fiber** 2g, **Sodium** 291mg

2 cans (5 ounces each) chunk white
    tuna in water, drained
2 tablespoons light ranch dressing
¼ cup peeled, diced cucumber
¼ cup diced celery

¼ cup diced carrot
1 small tomato, cut into 8 thin slices
2 toasted whole wheat English
    muffins, split
2 teaspoons fresh chopped dill

1. Combine tuna, dressing, cucumber, celery and carrot in medium bowl.

2. Place 2 tomato slices on each English muffin half. Top each evenly with tuna mixture and dill.

Makes 4 servings (1 open-faced sandwich per serving)

Dietary Exchanges: ½ Bread/Starch, 2 Vegetable, 2 Meat

Calories 188, **Total Fat** 5g, **Saturated Fat** 1g, **Protein** 20g, **Carbohydrates** 16g, **Cholesterol** 31mg, **Dietary Fiber** 3g, **Sodium** 507mg

July 10

Discuss with your doctor your goal for your A1c results. The American Diabetes Association recommends a goal of less than seven percent. Don't be upset if your result doesn't improve very quickly—it can take months to see significant changes. And be wary of comparing numbers from different laboratories.

July 8

Myth or Fact? A product labeled "sugar free" will always contain fewer carbohydrates than the regular version of the product.

Myth. A food labeled "sugar free" may not be lower in carbohydrates (or calories, for that matter). In fact, in the context of labeling, "sugar free" just means that a product contains less than .5 gram of sucrose, that is, cane or table sugar. Fructose or other sweeteners can still be added.

July 9

Your doctor may recommend periodic A1c (also known as HbA1c) tests. Why, if you're already testing your blood glucose levels with a meter? It's because the A1c test gives your doctor a good idea of your blood glucose level over recent months—it gives more than just a snapshot. Comparing the results of an A1c test with the averages you compile on your own can also help you determine whether your meter is accurate.